"The glycemic index is a useful tool which may have a broad spectrum of applications, from the maintenance of fuel supply during exercise to the control of blood glucose levels in diabetics. Low glycemic index foods may prove to have beneficial health effects for all of us in the long term. *The Glucose Revolution* is a user-friendly, easy-to-read overview of all that you need to know about the glycemic index. This book represents a balanced account of the importance of the glycemic index based on sound scientific evidence."

—JAMES HILL, PH.D., Director, Center for Human Nutrition, University of Colorado Health Sciences Center

"*The New Glucose Revolution* summarizes much of the recent development of dietary glycemic index and load in a highly readable format. The authors are able researchers and respected leaders in the nutrition field. Much that is discussed in this book draws directly from their years of experimental and observational research. The focus on dietary intervention and prevention strategies in everyday eating is an especially laudable feature of this book. I recommend this book most highly as an indispensable source of good nutrition."

—SIMIN LIU, M.D., SC.D., Assistant Professor, Department of Epidemiology, Harvard School of Public Health

"As a coach of elite amateur and professional athletes, I know how critical the glycemic index is to sports performance. *The New Glucose Revolution* provides the serious athlete with the basic tools necessary for getting the training table right."

—JOE FRIEL, coach, author, consultant

Other Glucose Revolution & New Glucose Revolution Titles

The New Glucose Revolution: The Authoritative Guide to the Glycemic Index—the Dietary Solution for Lifelong Health

The Glucose Revolution Life Plan

What Makes My Blood Glucose Go Up ... And Down? And 101 Other Frequently Asked Questions about Your Blood Glucose Levels

The New Glucose Revolution Complete Guide to Glycemic Index Values

The New Glucose Revolution Pocket Guide to the Top 100 Low GI Foods

The New Glucose Revolution Pocket Guide to Diabetes

The New Glucose Revolution Pocket Guide to Losing Weight

The New Glucose Revolution Pocket Guide to the Metabolic Syndrome and Your Heart

■

The Glucose Revolution Pocket Guide to Sugar and Energy

The Glucose Revolution Pocket Guide to the Glycemic Index and Healthy Kids

The Glucose Revolution Pocket Guide to Children with Type 1 Diabetes

■

FORTHCOMING

The New Glucose Revolution Life Plan

The New Glucose Revolution Pocket Guide to Healthy Kids

The New Glucose Revolution Pocket Guide to Childhood Diabetes

The New Glucose Revolution Pocket Guide to Sugar and Energy

The New Glucose Revolution Guide to Managing PCOS

The NEW GLUCOSE *Revolution*

POCKET GUIDE TO

PEAK PERFORMANCE

Helen O'Connor, B.Sc., Dip. N.D., Ph.D.
Jennie Brand-Miller, Ph.D.
Stephen Colagiuri, M.D.
Kaye Foster-Powell, M. Nutr. & Diet.

Marlowe & Company
New York

THE NEW GLUCOSE REVOLUTION POCKET GUIDE TO PEAK PERFORMANCE

Published by
Marlowe & Company
An Imprint of Avalon Publishing Group Incorporated
245 West 17th Street • 11th Floor
New York, NY 10011

This edition published in somewhat different form in Australia in 2003
under the title *The New Glucose Revolution Peak Performance* by Hodder
Headline Australia Pty Limited. This edition published by arrangement
with Hodder Headline Australia Pty Limited.

The GI logo is a trademark of the University of Sydney in Australia
and other countries. A food product carrying this logo is nutritious and
has been tested for its GI by an accredited laboratory.

Library of Congress Cataloging-in-Publication Data

The new glucose revolution pocket guide to peak performance / Helen
O'Connor ... [et al.].
p. cm.
Includes bbliographical references.
ISBN 1-56924-447-2
1. Athletes—Nutrition. 2. Glycemic index. I. O'Connor, Helen.
TX361.A8.N49 2003
613.2'024'796—dc21   2003059905

9 8 7 6 5 4 3 2 1

Designed by Pauline Neuwirth, Neuwirth & Associates, Inc.
Printed in the United States of America
Distributed by Publishers Group West

CONTENTS

PREFACE

THE NEW GLUCOSE REVOLUTION is the definitive, all-in-one guide to the glycemic index. Now we have written this pocket guide to show you how the glycemic index (GI) can help you enhance your sports performance—whether you're a weekend warrior or a serious athlete.

The Glucose Revolution Pocket Guide to Peak Performance offers more in-depth information about using the glycemic index to boost your athletic performance than we had room to include in *The New Glucose Revolution*. Much new information appears in this book that is not in *The New Glucose Revolution*, including the questions most frequently asked by athletes about the glycemic index; recommendations about what to eat before a competition, during an event, and for a quick recovery; and success stories profiling athletes who have gained the winning edge by eating low—and high—GI foods at the appropriate times.

This book was written to be read alongside *The New Glucose Revolution*, so in the event you haven't already consulted that book, please be sure to do so, for a more comprehensive discussion of the glycemic index and all its uses.

1

HOW THIS BOOK
CAN HELP YOU

*S*PORTS NUTRITION IS a new and dynamic science dedicated to unraveling the key nutrition factors that boost sports performance. What you eat does make a difference to your performance. The trick is getting into the right eating routine, keeping up to date, and ignoring the confusing nutrition myths that abound.

This book looks at a key factor: the glycemic index (or GI). Australian researchers were the first to see the potential in applying the glycemic index to athletes' diets to enhance sports performance, and now trainers, registered dietitians, and athletes the world over are using the glycemic index to give them a competitive edge. We'll discuss the glycemic index in more detail in chapters 5 and 6.

This guide shows you how to use the glycemic index in your own diet to boost your sports performance. When you pop this pocket book into your training bag, you'll have:

- a quick quiz to help you assess your current eating habits
- refueling tips at your fingertips
- case studies that provide you with fun, easy, and practical ways to eat your way to better performance
- GI tables of foods, including sports drinks, plus their fat and carbohydrate count

■

**What you eat does make a difference
to your sports performance.**

■

◀ 2 ▶

IS YOUR DIET FIT FOR PEAK PERFORMANCE?

*D*O YOU THINK your current diet supplies you with the nutrients you need to perform at your best? Let's put it to the test. Take the following diet fitness quiz and see how well you score. It's a good idea to use this quiz regularly to pick up on areas where you may need to improve your diet.

1. *Circle "Yes" or "No" below each quiz item.*

Eating patterns

▶ I eat at least 3 meals a day with no longer than 5 hours in between.
Yes / No

Carbohydrate checker

▶ I eat at least 4 slices of bread each day (1 roll = 2 slices of bread).
Yes / No

▶ I eat at least 1 cup of breakfast cereal each day or
an extra slice of bread.
Yes / No

▶ I usually eat 2 or more pieces of fruit each day.
Yes / No

▶ I eat at least 5 different vegetables or have a large
salad most days.
Yes / No

▶ I include carbohydrates like pasta, rice, and potato
in my diet each day.
Yes / No

Protein checker

▶ I eat at least 1 and usually 2 servings of meat or
meat alternatives (poultry, seafood, eggs, dried
peas, beans, or nuts) each day.
Yes / No

Fat checker

▶ I spread butter or margarine thinly on bread or
use none at all.
Yes / No

▶ I eat fried food no more than once per week.
Yes / No

▶ I use polyunsaturated or monounsaturated oil
(canola or olive) for cooking. (Circle yes if you
never fry in oil or fat.)
Yes / No

▶ I avoid oil-based dressings on salads.
Yes / No

▶ I use reduced-fat or low-fat dairy products.
Yes / No

▶ I cut the fat off meat and take the skin off chicken.
  Yes / *No*

▶ I eat fatty snacks such as chocolate, chips, biscuits, or rich desserts/cakes, etc., no more than twice a week.
  Yes / *No*

▶ I eat fast or take-out food no more than once per week.
  Yes / *No*

Iron checker

▶ I eat lean red meat at least 3 times per week or 2 servings of white meat daily or, for vegetarians, include at least 1 or 2 cups of dried peas and beans (such as lentils, soy beans, chickpeas) daily.
  Yes / *No*

▶ I include a vitamin C source with meals based on bread, cereals, fruit, and vegetables to assist the iron absorption in these plant sources of iron.
  Yes / *No*

Calcium checker

▶ I eat at least 3 servings of dairy food or soy milk alternative each day (1 serving = 8 ounces milk or fortified soy milk; 1-ounce slice of hard cheese; 8 ounces yogurt).
  Yes / *No*

Fluids

▶ I drink fluids regularly before, during, and after exercise.
  Yes / *No*

Alcohol

- ◗ When I drink alcohol, I usually drink no more than is recommended for the safe driving limit. (Circle "Yes" if you don't drink alcohol.)

  Yes / No

2. *Score 1 point for every "Yes" answer.*

Scoring scale

18–20: Excellent

15–17: Room for improvement

12–14: Just made it

0–12: Poor

Note: *Very* active people will need to eat more breads, cereals, and fruit than we have outlined on this quiz, but to stay healthy no one should be eating less. The food amounts in this quiz are devised for adults—not children or adolescents. (Adapted from *The Taste of Fitness* by Helen O'Connor and Donna Hay.)

◀ 3 ▶

SPORTS NUTRITION
IN A NUTSHELL

To PERFORM AT its best, your body needs the right type of fuel. No matter what your sport, carbohydrates are the best fuel for you. High-carbohydrate foods help enhance stamina and prevent fatigue. These types of food include breakfast cereals, bread, rice, pasta, fruit, and vegetables (especially starchy vegetables like new potatoes, corn, and dried peas and beans). Sugars found in table sugar, honey, jam, and candy are also useful sources of carbohydrate for active people.

LOW-FAT EATING

Fats are an essential part of your diet. A low to moderate fat intake helps active people maintain a lean physique. But eating the best types of fat and avoiding excessive fat intake is important for good health as well as best performance. The best types of fats for cooking include monounsaturated fats such as olive and canola oil and polyunsaturated fats such as sunflower and safflower oil. Watch out for the saturated fats found in many fast foods, as well as butter, cream, and the visible fat on meat.

It's never to late to start reducing the amount of fat in your diet. Here's how:

- cut the fat off meat (or use lean cuts)
- remove the skin from chicken
- use minimal amounts of fat in cooking, or substitute with vegetable sprays
- use nonstick cookware

The amount of fat you need depends on your daily fuel requirements. For good health and weight maintenance we have included the following general guidelines. (five grams fat is equivalent to about 1 teaspoon mono- or polyunsaturated oil.)

Low-fat diets	30 to 40 g fat per day
Most women and children	30 to 50 g fat per day
Most men	40 to 60 g fat per day
Teenagers and active adults	70 g fat per day
Larger and very active athletes/workers	80 to 100 g fat per day

Fat is a seemingly invisible ingredient in many foods. Use a fat counter to help you identify some of the sources of fat in your diet. Keep a food record for a week and calculate your personal fat intake using the counter. It may surprise you! (Comprehensive fat counters are readily available from bookstores and supermarkets.)

Are You Really Choosing Low-Fat?

THERE'S A TRICK to food labels that it is worth being aware of when shopping for low-fat foods. These food-labeling specification guidelines were enacted by the United States Department of Agriculture (USDA) in 1994:

Free: Contains a tiny or insignificant amount of fat, cholesterol, sodium, sugar, or calories; less than 0.5 grams (g) of fat per serving.

Low fat: Contains no more than 3 g of fat per serving.

Reduced/Less/Fewer: These diet products must contain 25 percent less of a nutrient or calories than the regular product.

Light/Lite: These diet products contain ⅓ fewer calories than, or ½ the fat of, the original product.

Lean: Meats claiming this contain less than 10 g of fat, 4 g of saturated fat, and 95 milligrams (mg) of cholesterol per serving.

Extra lean: These meats have less than 5 g of fat, 2 g of saturated fat, 95 mg of cholesterol.

■

A balanced diet
contains a wide
variety of low-fat foods.

■

DON'T FORGET PROTEIN

Athletes in heavy training have increased protein needs. Protein balance depends on the individual, but you generally need at least two or three servings a day. Some athletes forget to include enough protein in their diets, while bodybuilders often consume more protein than their bodies need. Good sources of protein include lean meat, poultry, fish and seafood, eggs, milk, cheese, and yogurt. Dried peas, beans, and nuts are the best vegetable sources. Bread and cereals provide smaller, but still useful, amounts of protein.

FLUIDS

The human body is 70 percent water. During exercise you lose some of this water as sweat. If you don't replace it, you will become dehydrated and your body will overheat—like a car without water in its radiator.

- Small fluid losses decrease mental and physical performance.
- Large fluid losses can result in dehydration and are life-threatening!

During exercise, thirst isn't a good indicator of how much fluid your body needs, so don't use that as your guide. Be sure to drink more than your thirst dictates. Every pound lost during exercise approximates a pint of sweat losses to be replaced.

■

During exercise, thirst is not a good indicator of your fluid needs.

■

WHAT TO DRINK DURING EXERCISE

It's hard to know exactly what to drink when you're working out, because there are so many options. From water to sports drinks to fruit juice, here are some guidelines to help quench your thirst:

▶ Water replaces lost fluids adequately in many situations.

▶ Sports and electrolyte drinks are absorbed into the bloodstream faster than water. In addition to replacing carbohydrates and electrolytes, they taste good, which encourages you to drink more. (See chapter 10 on page 49 for more on sports drinks.) The A to Z table of foods (chapter 19 on page 97) gives the GI value of the sports drink Gatorade.

▶ Soft drinks and fruit juice empty from the stomach more slowly than sports drinks or water and aren't suitable fluid replacers during exercise.

Note: Be careful with caffeine-containing beverages while exercising. The caffeine increases urine production, which can make you dehydrated.

■

Adequate fluid replacement
during exercise enhances performance
and prevents heat stress.

■

SPECIAL NUTRIENT CONSIDERATIONS

Of course, everyone—athletes and non-athletes alike—
needs to make sure they're eating right and getting adequate amounts of important nutrients. But athletes,
laborers, and avid exercisers need to be especially careful to take in the appropriate amounts of vitamins, minerals, and other nutrients to perform better and longer,
without ill effects.

Best Sources of Iron

(ranked from highest to lowest):
**** Red meats and liver
*** White meats and seafood
** Dried peas and beans (baked beans, soy beans)
* Bread, cereals, and some vegetables

Iron

Iron deficiency is common in athletes, particularly
female athletes, vegetarians, and those participating in
strenuous training programs, such as endurance athletes. Many athletes don't consume adequate iron in

their daily diets and may take in too much caffeine or tannin (in tea), which binds up the available iron and reduces its absorption. The best sources of iron are red meats and liver. Plant sources contain lower amounts of iron, and the iron isn't absorbed as well. And the iron in iron supplements is also less well absorbed than the iron in red meat.

Did You Know?

INCLUDING VITAMIN C-RICH fruits and vegetables in a meal improves the absorption of iron from plant sources (e.g., bread, cereals, vegetables, fruit). Drinking a glass of orange juice with your cereal in the morning will increase the amount of iron absorbed from this meal.

Calcium

Calcium is important for bone development in young people and for bone maintenance in adults. Getting enough calcium and participating in weight-bearing exercise throughout life is essential to build—then maintain—optimal bone strength for both males and females.

■

**Calcium is important
for bone development in the young
and for bone maintenance in adults.**

■

In females, regular strenuous exercise, usually accompanied by factors such as fat loss, strict dieting, or stress, can precipitate menstrual cycle interruptions. An irregular or absent menstrual cycle may result in a reduced level of the hormone estrogen, which is vital for maintaining calcium levels in bone and for enhancing calcium absorption. If you have experienced menstrual irregularities for longer than six months, you should see a doctor to help determine the cause. Athletes with very infrequent or absent menstrual cycles should have extra calcium in the range of 1,000 to 1,500 mg a day. This won't prevent bone loss, but may help to slow down the rate of loss.

NUTRITIONAL SUPPLEMENTS

Companies spend lots of money promoting nutritional supplements for active people and athletes. Just watch out for supplements with no scientific basis to the claims. If in doubt, ask a sports dietitian for help. (See page 134 for information on locating a registered dietitian near you.) Some supplements are beneficial in certain circumstances.

- You may need iron or calcium supplements if you consume inadequate amounts of these minerals or if you have a deficiency.
- You might also benefit from supplements such as sports drinks, liquid meals, and carbohydrate loaders, not because they provide anything magical, but because they package energy and carbohydrate in a convenient and easy-to-consume form.

They're especially useful to athletes who need an easily digested fuel on the run.

▶ Sports bars and carbohydrate gels (available in sports and bike shops) are in a similar category to sports drinks.

▶ Herbal supplements, amino acids, and fat burners: unfortunately, solid evidence for these supplements is lacking. In many cases, scientific studies have shown absolutely no effect.

▶ Always make sure that any supplements you take are safe and drug-free. Some herbal supplements have actually caused some athletes to register "positive" on drug tests. Check with your sport's governing body to make sure the herb or medicine that you're taking is approved.

COMPETITION EATING

Eating for competing is discussed in detail later in this book. Look under the following topics:

▶ Pre-competition meal guidelines (page 44)
▶ Glycogen loading (page 42)
▶ Recovery after exercise (page 54)
▶ The case for high-GI foods (page 53)
▶ Refueling during an event (page 49)

If you want to find out about eating for competing in greater depth, consult a sports dietitian.

■

**Whether you are one of the elite
or a weekend warrior,
the right diet can give you
the winning edge.**

■

◀ 4 ▶

ENERGY-CHARGE YOUR BODY WITH CARBOHYDRATE

*C*ARBOHYDRATE CIRCULATES IN your body as glucose in the blood (blood sugar) and is stored as glycogen in the liver and muscles. When glycogen stores are depleted, fatigue sets in and performance suffers. Your body uses glucose to fuel movement and activity. Just as high-speed cars require regular gasoline fill-ups, active bodies need a regular supply of carbohydrate to fill up glycogen stores.

Carbohydrate is the human body's favorite energy source for physical activity—especially for high-intensity exercise. But your body's carbohydrate stores are small and need regular replenishing, generally every four to five hours.

Athletes feel tired and lethargic when they don't consume enough carbohydrate to meet their daily needs. When this happens and the glycogen in the muscles is depleted, fatigue sets in. That's when your muscles feel heavy and your pace slows. "Hitting the wall," an expression used by endurance athletes, describes the feeling when glycogen stores are almost exhausted.

■

Active bodies need a regular supply of carbohydrate to fill up their glycogen stores.

■

LOW BLOOD SUGAR OR "HYPOGLYCEMIA"

People who work out can also experience a type of fatigue related to the carbohydrate levels in their blood. It is possible for your muscle glycogen levels to be adequate while the blood-sugar levels, controlled by the liver, fall. Low blood sugar (also known as "hypoglycemia") occurs when you exercise in the morning before eating, or exercise hard after skipping a meal.

■

To maintain energy levels, athletes must consume enough carbohydrate to keep pace with their muscle glycogen needs and keep up a regular intake of carbohydrate to maintain blood-sugar levels.

■

EARLY MORNING EXERCISE

If you exercise strenuously early in the morning, it's a good idea to have some carbohydrate before training or take some with you to have on the run. Most people have enough liver glycogen to fuel low-intensity, short-duration (less than one hour) exercise sessions. If you simply want to delay eating until after your light early morning walk, it's not a problem. However, eating before and/or during a strenuous cycling session makes good sense.

THREE EASY STEPS TO ESTIMATE YOUR DAILY CARBOHYDRATE NEEDS

It's difficult to put an exact figure on anyone's carbohydrate needs. Use the table on pages 34–35 as a rough guide and ask a sports dietitian for help if you're still unsure.

Step 1. Weigh yourself naked or in minimal clothing in kilograms. To do this, multiply your weight in pounds by 2.2. (Remember: no shoes or belts with heavy buckles!)

Step 2. Multiply your body weight by your activity level factor (see table on pages 34–35). This total gives you the target carbohydrate intake in grams that you must consume each day to meet your carbohydrate needs.

Step 3. Keep a food record for a few days and calculate your carbohydrate intake (use a carbohydrate counter such as the one in the A to Z GI values table at the end of this book). Compare your actual carbohydrate intake with the target value you calculated. If it is far below the carbohydrate target, you have some serious carb eating to do. If you're within 50 grams, or even

a little over, your carbohydrate target, that's fine. Use
the carbohydrate counter to help you plan a higher carb
intake. Remember, this is a rough estimate; you may
need a little more or less carbohydrate, depending on
how you feel.

◀ 5 ▶

WHICH CARBOHYDRATE FOODS ARE BEST?

CARBOHYDRATE FOODS INCLUDE breads, breakfast cereals, rice, pasta, fruit, and vegetables, especially starchy vegetables such as new potatoes, corn, and dried peas and beans. There are smaller amounts of carbohydrate in dairy foods and in processed foods containing sugars. The carbohydrate foods give you a range of nutrients essential for good health. When you're establishing the overall balance of your diet, it is important to consume more of the carbohydrate foods that contain a high proportion of nutrients (we call these "nutrient-dense") than those without additional vitamins and minerals.

Many active people, especially athletes in heavy training who eat large volumes of food, easily meet their daily nutrient requirements. Their carbohydrate needs, however, are sometimes so high, they simply can't manage the volume they need to eat! Liquid meals or carbohydrate supplements can help these athletes meet their energy needs in a less "bulky" way.

■

Today, there's another vital consideration in selecting
carbohydrate foods to boost your sports performance.
It is the glycemic index value of a food.

■

CARBOHYDRATES
AND THE GLYCEMIC INDEX

Carbohydrates and carbohydrate foods that break down
quickly during digestion have the highest GI values. The
blood-glucose, or sugar, response is fast and high. In
other words, the glucose in the bloodstream increases
rapidly. Conversely, carbohydrates that break down slowly,
releasing glucose gradually into the bloodstream, have
low GI values. An analogy might be the popular fable of
the tortoise and the hare. The hare, just like high-GI
foods, speeds away full steam ahead but loses the race to
the tortoise, with his slow and steady pace. Similarly,
slow and steady low-GI foods produce a smooth blood-
sugar curve without wild fluctuations.

For most people most of the time, foods with low GI
values have advantages over those with high GI values.
Figure 1 shows the effect of slow and fast carbohydrate
on blood-sugar levels.

The substance that produces the greatest rise in
blood-sugar levels is pure glucose itself. All other foods
have less effect when fed in equal amounts of carbohydrate. The GI value of pure glucose is set at 100, and
every other food is ranked on a scale from 0 to 100
according to its actual effect on blood-sugar levels.

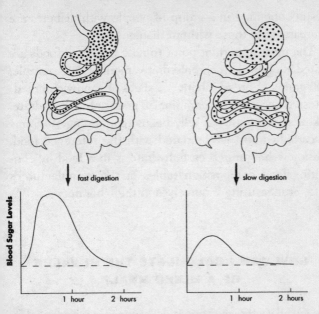

Figure 1. Slow and fast carbohydrate digestion and the consequent levels of sugar in the blood.

The GI value of a food cannot be predicted from its composition or the GI values of related foods. To test the glycemic index, you need real people and real foods. We describe how the GI value of a food is measured in the following chapter. There is no easy, inexpensive substitute test. Scientists always follow standardized methods so that results from one group of people can be directly compared with those of another group.

In total, eight to ten people need to be tested, and the GI value of the food is the average value of the group. We know this average figure is reproducible and that a different group of volunteers will produce a similar result.

Results obtained in a group of people with diabetes are comparable to those without diabetes.

The most important point to note is that all foods are tested in equivalent carbohydrate amounts. For example, 100 grams of bread (about 3½ slices of sandwich bread) is tested because this contains 50 grams of carbohydrate. Likewise, 60 grams of jelly beans (containing 50 grams of carbohydrate) is compared with the reference food. We know how much carbohydrate is in a food by consulting food composition tables or the manufacturer's data, or measuring it ourselves in the laboratory.

HOW CAN I CALCULATE THE GI VALUE OF A MIXED MEAL?

You calculate the glycemic index value of a mixed meal by averaging the GI value of the different carbohydrate foods in the meal. Let's use hummus on toast as an example: regular white bread has a GI value of 70 and hummus has a GI value of 42. If equal amounts of carbohydrate come from the hummus and the bread, then you add the GI values and divide by two: $(70 + 42)/2 = 56$.

Let's say the meal contained one-quarter of the carbohydrate from hummus to three-quarters of the carbohydrate from bread; then 25 percent of the GI value for hummus would be added to 75 percent of the GI value for bread. The following shows how to calculate this.

$$42 \times .25 \quad = 10.5$$
$$70 \times .75 \quad = 52.5$$
$$\text{GI value} \quad = 10.5 + 52.5 = 63$$

But you really don't need to do calculations. All you need to remember is:

Low GI + High GI = Intermediate GI

6

UNDERSTANDING THE GLYCEMIC INDEX

THE GI IS a scientifically validated tool in the dietary management of diabetes, weight reduction, and athletic performance.

Originally, research into the glycemic index of foods was inspired by the desire to identify the best foods for people with diabetes. But scientists are now discovering that the glycemic index has positive implications for everyone.

■

The GI is a ranking of foods based on their overall effect on blood-glucose levels

■

HOW THE GLYCEMIC INDEX CAME TO BE

The glycemic index concept was first developed in 1981 by Dr. David Jenkins, a professor of nutrition at the University of Toronto, Canada, to help determine which foods were best for people with diabetes. At that time, the diet for people with diabetes was based on a system of carbohydrate exchanges, which assumed that all carbohydrate foods produced the same effect on blood-glucose levels, even though earlier studies had already proven this was not correct. Jenkins was one of the first people to question this assumption and investigate how real foods behave in the bodies of real people.

Since then, scientists, including the authors of this book, have tested the effect of many foods on blood-glucose levels, and clinical studies in the United Kingdom, France, Italy, Australia, and Canada have all proven without doubt the value of the glycemic index.

The GI value of foods is simply a ranking of carbohydrates in foods according to their immediate impact on blood-glucose levels. Because carbohydrates have the greatest effect on blood-sugar levels, the glycemic index focuses on these foods. And why should you be concerned about blood-sugar levels? Because our blood-sugar level at any given time determines how much energy we have, how mentally clear we are, and how hungry we feel.

Today we know the GI values of hundreds of different food items that have been tested following the standardized method. We have included many of these values in the tables at the back of this book, but for more detailed information you should consult *The New Glucose Revolution* or *The New Glucose Revolution Complete Guide to Glycemic Index Values*.

THE KEY IS THE RATE OF DIGESTION

Foods containing carbohydrates that break down quickly during digestion have the highest GI values. The blood-glucose response is fast and high (in other words, the glucose in the bloodstream increases rapidly). Conversely, foods that contain carbohydrates that break down slowly, releasing glucose gradually into the bloodstream, have low GI values.

For most people most of the time, foods with low GI values have advantages over those with high GI values. This is especially true for people trying to control their weight (or lose weight).

The higher the GI value of a food, the higher the blood-glucose levels after eating that food. Instant white rice (GI value 87) and baked potatoes (GI value 85) have very high GI values, meaning their effect on blood-glucose levels is almost as high as that of an equal amount of pure glucose (yes, you read it correctly).

Figure 2 shows the blood-glucose response to potatoes compared with pure glucose. Foods with a low GI value (such as lentils at 29) show a flatter blood-glucose response when eaten, as shown in Figure 3. The peak blood-glucose level is lower and the return to the more normal baseline levels is slower than with a high-GI food.

■

GI RANGES
Low GI value = 55 or less
Intermediate GI value = 56 to 69
High GI value = 70 or more

▪

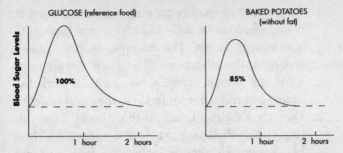

Figure 2. The effect of pure glucose (50 g) and baked potatoes without fat (50 g carbohydrate portion) on blood-glucose levels.

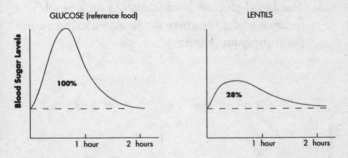

Figure 3. The effect of pure glucose (50 g) and lentils (50 g carbohydrate portion) on blood-glucose levels.

HOW WE MEASURE THE GLUCEMIC INDEX

Pure glucose produces the greatest rise in blood-glucose levels. Most foods have less effect when fed in equal carbohydrate quantities. The GI value of pure glucose is set at 100 and every other food is ranked on a scale from 0 to 100 according to its actual effect on blood-glucose levels.

1. An amount of food containing a standard amount of carbohydrate (usually 25 or 50 grams) is given to a volunteer to eat. For example, to test cooked spaghetti, the volunteer will be given 200 grams of spaghetti, which supplies 50 grams of carbohydrate (determined from food-composition tables).

2. Over the next two hours (or three hours if the volunteer has diabetes), we take a sample of their blood every 15 minutes during the first hour and thereafter every 30 minutes. The blood-glucose level of these blood samples is measured in the laboratory and recorded.

3. The blood-glucose level is plotted on a graph and the area under the curve is calculated using a computer program (Figure 4).

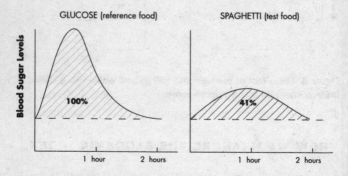

Figure 4. Measuring the GI value of a food.
The test food and the reference food must contain the same amount of carbohydrate. The usual dose is 50 grams, but sometimes 25 grams is used when the portion size would otherwise be too large. Even smaller doses, such as 15 grams, have been used. The GI value is much the same whatever the dose, because the GI number is simply a relative measure of carbohydrate quality.

4. The volunteer's response to spaghetti (or whatever food is being tested) is compared with his or her blood-glucose response to 50 grams of pure glucose (the reference food).

5. The reference food is tested on two or three separate occasions and an average value is calculated. This is done to reduce the effect of day-to-day variation in blood-glucose responses.

6. The average GI value found in eight to ten people is the GI value of that food.

Key Factors That Influence the Glycemic Index

■ **Cooking methods**
Cooking and processing increases the GI value of a food because it increases the swelling of the starch molecules in the food. Rice is one example.

■ **Physical form of the food**
An intact fibrous coat, such as that on whole grains and legumes, acts as a physical barrier and slows down digestion, lowering a food's GI value. Beans, barley, and whole-grain pumpernickel are examples.

■ **Type of starch**
There are two types of starch in foods, amylose and amylopectin. The more amylose starch a food contains, the lower the GI value.

■ **Particle size**
The smaller the particle size, the easier it is for water and enzymes to penetrate. This is why enriched wheat

continued

flour (which is a highly processed, finely milled flour) has a high GI value, while stone-ground flour, with larger particles, has a lower GI value.

■ Fiber

Viscous, soluble fibers, such as those found in rolled oats and apples, slow down digestion and lower a food's GI value.

■ Sugar

The presence of sugar, as well as the type of sugar, will influence a food's GI value. Fruits with a low GI value, such as apples and oranges, are high in fructose. The presence of sugar also will restrict gelatinization (or swelling) of starch that is present in a food by binding with the water in the food. So some cookies and breakfast cereals that contain sugar may have relatively low GI values.

■ Acidity

Acids in foods slow down stomach emptying, thereby slowing the rate at which the starch can be digested. Vinegar, lemon juice, lime juice, salad dressings, pickled vegetables, and sourdough bread are good examples.

■ Fat

Fat slows down the rate of stomach emptying, thereby slowing the digestion of the starch. For example, potato chips have a lower GI value than boiled potatoes.

TRICKY TWINS

Circle the food in each of the following pairs that you think will have the lower GI value.

Rice	Kellogg's Rice Krispies™
Corn	Corn flakes
Baked potatoes	French fries
Toasted muesli	Untoasted muesli
Whole-grain bread	Whole-wheat bread

Answers: Rice, corn, baked potatoes, toasted muesli, whole-grain bread (depending on the brand).

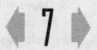

WHAT'S YOUR
ACTIVITY LEVEL?

$\mathcal{T}$HE AMOUNT OF carbohydrate you need depends on your weight and activity level. Below, we offer step-by-step guidelines to help you calculate your needs.

ACTIVITY LEVEL	GRAMS OF CARBOHYDRATE PER KG BODY WEIGHT PER DAY
Light: Walking, light/easy swimming or cycling; low-impact /easy beat aerobic dance Less than 1 hour per day	4–5
Light–moderate: Intermediate aerobic dance class; easy jog; non-competitive tennis (3 sets); volleyball 1 hour per day	5–6
Moderate: 1-hour run; serious training for recreational/competition sports such as soccer, basketball, squash 1–2 hours per day	6–7

ACTIVITY LEVEL	GRAMS OF CARBOHYDRATE PER KG BODY WEIGHT PER DAY
Moderate–heavy: Most professional/ elite training for competitive sport such as swimming, tennis, football, distance running (except marathons) 2–4 hours per day	7–8
Heavy: Training for Ironman events; marathon running/swimming; Olympic distance triathlon More than 4 hours per day	8–10

■ Activity levels refer to the intensity as well as the duration of the activity.
■ Time refers to the amount of time you are physically active during training, not the amount of time at training.
■ Body weight refers to ideal or healthy body weight.

Here's an example of how the numbers add up for one athlete.

Jessica's Carbohydrate Needs

Step 1. Weight   128 lbs. (58 kg)

Step 2. Activity   Moderate level (training for mid-distance fun runs such as 5 or 10Ks—recreational level)
Requires 6–7 g of carbohydrate per kilogram per day
Target carbohydrate level is:
  6 x 58 = 348 g per day to 7 x 58 = 406 g per day
348–406 g per day

Step 3.   Food record

Jessica's Food Record

MEAL	CARBOHYDRATE COUNT (g)
Breakfast	
1 cup of bran flakes	36
½ cup of milk	6
1 slice of white toast with butter	14
4 oz. no-sugar-added fruit juice	18
Snack	
1 medium banana	24

MEAL	CARBOHYDRATE COUNT (g)
Lunch	
1 cheese and tomato sandwich on white bread	28
6 oz. light fruit yogurt	11
1 glass water	0
Snack	
Kavli™ All Natural Whole Grain	
Crispbread, 4 wafers, with peanut butter	13
1 orange	11
Dinner	
1 small piece of steak	0
1 medium potato	30
½ cup of mixed frozen vegetables	12
½ cup low-fat ice cream	9
Snack	
4 Nabisco Social Tea biscuits™	13
Total carbohydrate	**225**

Jessica's carbohydrate count is way below target.

To boost Jessica's carbohydrate **intake, add:**	
1 extra piece of toast at breakfast	14
1 cup split pea soup and 1 cup natural	
applesauce at lunch	54
1 cup cooked brown rice with dinner and increase	
mixed vegetables to 1 cup	57
1 bread roll with dinner	14
6 Nabisco Social Tea biscuits™	19
Grand total boosted with the extra carbohydrate foods	**383 g**

This is in the middle of the recommended range for Jessica's weight and activity level. Depending on how she feels, she may need to make slight adjustments depending on variations in the intensity and duration of her training program.

8

USING THE GLYCEMIC INDEX TO BOOST SPORTS PERFORMANCE

THERE ARE SEVERAL applications of the glycemic index to sports performance. Sometimes it will be best to choose a high-GI food, while at other times, a low-GI food may be more beneficial. Choosing one type of food over another depends on what you want to accomplish.

To date, most work on the glycemic index and sports performance has concentrated on competition eating and recovery. Over the past few years, however, several studies suggest that eating low- to moderate-GI foods prior to an event can prolong endurance. In fact, one study showed that time to exhaustion was 59 percent longer after athletes had eaten a meal with a low GI value!

A HIGH-CARBOHYDRATE DIET IS ESSENTIAL FOR PEAK ATHLETIC PERFORMANCE

A high-carbohydrate diet is a must for optimum athletic performance because it produces the largest stores of muscle glycogen. As we have previously described, the carbohydrate we eat is stored in the body in the form of glycogen in the muscles and liver. A small amount of carbohydrate (about 1 teaspoon) circulates as glucose in the blood. When you're exercising at a high intensity, your muscles rely on glycogen and glucose for fuel. Although the body can use fat when you're exercising at lower intensities, fat can't provide the fuel fast enough when you are working very hard. The larger your stores of glycogen and glucose, the longer you can go before fatigue sets in.

Unlike the fat stores in the body that can release almost unlimited amounts of fatty acids, the carbohydrate stores are small, and are fully depleted after two or three hours of strenuous exercise. It's also when blood-glucose concentrations begin to decline. If you continue to exercise at the same rate, blood glucose may drop to levels that interfere with brain function and cause disorientation and unconsciousness.

MISCONCEPTIONS ABOUT CARBOHYDRATES

Many athletes and coaches have misconceptions about carbohydrates that can affect athletic performance. In the past we were taught that simple carbohydrates (sugars) were digested and absorbed rapidly while complex carbohydrates (starches) were digested slowly. We assumed (completely incorrectly) that simple carbohydrates gave the most rapid rises in blood sugar while complex carbohydrates produced gradual rises. Unfortunately, these assumptions had no factual or scientific basis. Instead, they were based on structural considerations: smaller molecules, like sugars, were thought to be easier to digest than larger ones, such as starches. Even though incorrect, the seemingly logical nature of these assumptions meant that they were rarely questioned. Unfortunately, many people still think sugars are the best source of quick energy and that starches are our best source of sustained energy.

HOW CARBOHYDRATES CAN HELP

Scientific research has so far identified three key applications of the glycemic index to enhance performance.

1. A low-GI pre-event meal may enhance endurance in prolonged exercise.
2. High-GI foods or fluids during exercise help to maintain blood-sugar levels.
3. High-GI foods in the recovery phase after exercise help to accelerate glycogen replenishment.
4. Low-GI foods may help athletes and weekend warriors alike to feel full and satisfied after and between meals, and this may assist them in maintaining a more optimal weight or body-fat level for their sport.

Researchers at the University of Sydney in Australia found several years ago that a low-GI pre-event meal, at least one hour prior to endurance exercise, can delay fatigue by delivering greater amounts of carbohydrate to the muscles late in exercise. Look at it this way: the low-GI meal will still be digesting while you exercise—and providing an additional source of carbohydrate that you had long forgotten about. Slow-release (low-GI) carbohydrate is thought to be particularly useful for exercise of long duration when glycogen stores become limited. This is especially true when the ability to consume carbohydrate during the event is difficult or limited. Low-GI foods, because they are absorbed much more slowly, can be likened to a continuous injection of glucose during the event. This glucose "infusion" can boost energy when fatigue begins to set in.

Since the publication of the Australian research we mentioned above, there have been a number of other studies investigating the effect of eating low-GI meals before sporting events. Some of these studies show improved exercise performance, while others do not. When you're planning a pre-event meal, it's important to consider whether you'll be consuming the carbohydrate in food form (such as from bananas, sports bars, or carbohydrate gels) or in a sports drink, such as Gatorade™. As long as you eat carbohydrate before an event, the type of carbohydrate isn't as critical, because your blood-sugar levels will be maintained by the carbohydrate foods (usually high-GI; see page 50) you'll consume as you exercise.

Some athletes, though, may still benefit from a low-GI pre-event meal, if they have abnormal glucose tolerance or a tendency to experience low blood glucose, especially after eating meals with a high GI value (hypoglycemia). For these athletes, it's definitely worth experimenting with low-GI meals before exercise.

And before the event, choose low-GI foods that don't

contain too much fiber, since these foods produce excess gas. (Taking a bathroom pit stop during exercise can be very inconvenient!) Some good light and low-GI foods include:

- Pasta, cooked al dente;
- Some varieties of rice, including brown and Uncle Ben's Long Grain and Wild;
- Low-GI breads, such as those made from whole grains; and
- Certain breakfast cereals, including oatmeal.

Eat to Compete: Carbohydrate Loading

CARBOHYDRATE (OR GLYCOGEN) loading increases the body's store of glycogen in the liver and muscles. The extra glycogen provides additional fuel for endurance exercise when a normal glycogen store wouldn't be sufficient to maintain stamina.

To carbohydrate-load, athletes used to go through a glycogen-depletion phase that made the muscles "hungry" for glycogen. These early regimes were like torture, because athletes felt tired and irritable. This way of eating also made it difficult for athletes to maintain their motivation and concentration. After two or three days of the depletion phase, the athletes would then eat a high-carbohydrate diet, providing 9 to 10 g of carbohydrate for every kilogram of body weight, for another three days. During this time, glycogen stores increased by 200 to 300 percent.

In recent times, athletes have been using a modified carbohydrate-loading regimen that results in a similar glycogen store without the unpleasant "depletion" phase. Athletes simply taper training during the week prior to competition and consume a high-carbohydrate diet as described above for two to three days prior to competition.

Do you need to carbohydrate-load?

All athletes need an adequate normal store of carbohydrate to maximize performance. Carbohydrate loading, in its true sense, is needed only by endurance athletes exercising for longer than two hours, such as those people competing in triathlons, marathons, centuries, or other endurance events.

What about the glycemic index and carbohydrate loading?

At present there is insufficient scientific evidence to recommend a particular GI value for carbohydrate loading. It appears that high-GI diets may result in higher muscle-glycogen levels in non-athletes. It would seem reasonable to propose that a higher-GI diet may facilitate more effective glycogen loading, but further research is needed.

■

Carbohydrate loading increases
the body's store of glycogen,
which helps to prevent fatigue
during endurance events.

■

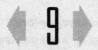

9

THE PRE-COMPETITION MEAL

*S*INCE THE PRE-COMPETITION meal has the potential to either make or break your performance on event day, what you eat should not be left to chance. Work on a dietary strategy using the following guidelines, then practice these principles before a training session to allow yourself time to fine-tune your pre-competition meal.

GUIDELINES

- Eat two to four hours before the event. This allows time for your pre-competition meal to empty from the stomach. Allow four hours for a larger meal.
- Make the meal high in carbohydrate for maximum energy.
- Fill up, don't overeat. Eat a comfortable amount of food.

▶ Keep your fat intake down for this meal, because fat slows digestion.

▶ Go for a moderate amount of protein. Fill up on carbohydrates instead.

▶ Aim for a moderate amount of fiber. Too much high-fiber food could cause bloating, diarrhea, and discomfort during the competition.

▶ Drink your meal. If you're too nervous, or you feel it's too early in the morning to eat, try a sports drink or liquid meal (such as Ensure Light or Super Shake) so that you can maintain your energy with liquid food.

▶ Practice. Experiment with different meals to find out what works best for you.

Ready?

On your mark

Remember, the pre-event meal won't work miracles if your training diet is inadequate. Make sure you are eating well generally, especially for the week leading up to competition.

Get set

Use these pre-competition guidelines to help you plan your pre-event meal.

Go!

During exercise, replace fluids and carbohydrates regularly as you go.

THE PRE-EVENT MEAL

Athletes like to eat foods that aren't too heavy or fibrous. If you want to try low-GI options, choose foods that are not too fibrous or gas-producing—taking a bathroom break during exercise can be very inconvenient! Suitable light and low-GI foods include pasta, some varieties of rice (Basmati, brown, Uncle Ben's Converted), low-GI breads (those with barley or whole grains) and some breakfast cereals (such as old-fashioned oats). For examples of low-GI foods, see the table on page 47.

The table shows the serving sizes of low-GI foods containing 50 or 75 grams of carbohydrate. (You can adjust the food amounts on the following list to make sure you're taking in the right amount of carbohydrate.) Keep in mind that you won't win any contests if your pre-event meal is jiggling around in your stomach (this will affect a runner more than a cyclist). So test the timing and amount of low-GI food during your training sessions. Then you'll be ready for the big day. Whatever you do, don't try it out for the first time on the day of the competition!

Serving Sizes of Low-GI Foods to Eat 1 to 2 Hours before the Event

FOOD	GLYCEMIC INDEX VALUE	SERVING SIZE = 50 G CARBOHYDRATE	SERVING SIZE = 75 G CARBOHYDRATE
Heavy grain breads, such as			4 to 5 slices
pumpernickel	41	3 slices (approx. 3 oz.)	(approx. 5 oz.)
Spaghetti, cooked	38	1½ cups (6 oz.)	2¼ cups (10 oz.)
Oatmeal, cooked	66	2½ cups (20 oz.)	3½ cups (32 oz.)
Baked beans	38	medium can (16 oz.)	1½ medium cans (24 oz.)
Fruit salad	approx. 50	2½ cups (approx. 16 oz.)	4 cups (28 oz.)
Yogurt (low-fat)	31	2 containers (16 oz.)	3 containers (24 oz.)
Apples	38	3 small or medium (16 oz.)	4 small (20 oz.)
Oranges	42	5 small (20 oz.)	7 small (32 oz.)
Dried apricots	30	¾ cup (4 oz.)	1⅛ cups (4 oz.)

Females who weigh about 110 pounds should aim to eat 50 grams of carbohydrate.

Males who weigh about 165 pounds should aim to eat 75 grams of carbohydrate.

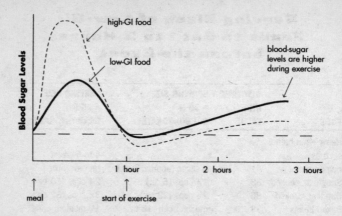

Figure 5. Comparison of the effect of low- and high-GI foods on blood-sugar levels during prolonged strenuous exercise. When a pre-event meal of lentils (low GI value) was compared with potatoes (high GI value), cyclists were able to continue cycling at a high intensity (65 percent of their peak aerobic capacity) for 20 minutes longer after eating the lentil meal. Their blood-sugar and insulin levels were significantly higher at the end of exercise, which indicated that the athletes were still absorbing carbohydrate from the small intestine even after 90 minutes of strenuous exercise.

◀ 10 ▶

DURING AN EVENT

*H*IGH-GI CARBOHYDRATE is the best choice to optimize performance, since the carbohydrate needs to be rapidly available to the muscle as a fuel source. Consuming carbohydrate "on the run" has been shown to delay fatigue because it provides energy to working muscles when the body's own stores of glycogen are low. This is especially true when exercise is prolonged and even glycogen loading cannot prepare the body for the carbohydrate needed to get through a long endurance event.

If you don't have sufficient carbohydrate in your training diet, supplementing carbohydrate during exercise helps you keep pace when your glycogen stores are low. Just remember: this isn't a quick fix to avoid a high-carbohydrate training diet! The body needs to obtain most of the carbs from glycogen stored in the muscles during exercise. Outside carbs are a great backup, but it's essential to prepare your body by eating a high-carb training diet each day.

The table below lists high-GI carbohydrates that are popular during exercise. Athletes usually tolerate sports electrolyte-replacement drinks better because they empty from the stomach more quickly.

High-GI Choices Suitable During Exercise

FOOD	GI	SERVING SIZE	CARBOHYDRATE (G)
Gatorade™	89	1 quart	60
Doughnut, cake type	76	2 doughnuts	46
Clif bar (cookies and cream)	101	2.4 oz.	34
Jelly beans	78	24 large (2½ oz.)	67
Rice cakes	82	7 cakes	49

■

Prolong your endurance by filling up on fluids and carbohydrate regularly throughout exercise.

□

Sports or electrolyte-replacement drinks are ideal because they encourage greater fluid consumption than water, enhance intestinal absorption of fluid, and provide carbohydrate while rehydrating your body at the same time. They are also less likely to cause gastrointestinal distress than solid foods.

The choice of solid or liquid carbohydrate during exercise is ultimately up to you. But with the current sports/electrolyte formulations providing an optimal, quickly absorbed source of carbohydrates, it is hard to look past this as a primary option. Many athletes choose a combination of sports drinks and comfortable solid foods they have tried while in training. During prolonged exercise, solid foods fill up that empty feeling in your stomach.

■

Use this book as a guide to start experimenting with different foods and fluids throughout training sessions. Discover for yourself what feels most comfortable and works best for you.

■

Many of the popular foods used during exercise over the years were adopted because they were convenient or easy to eat, rather than because they had a high GI value. The ever popular banana, for example, has an intermediate GI value. Eating a banana during exercise isn't wrong, but when the pace is really on and you want a fast energy supply, a more rapidly absorbing high-GI option would be better. In prolonged exercise, you should aim to consume 30 to 60 grams of carbohydrate per hour over the session or event.

During long events, a combination of comfortable foods (whatever their GI values), along with the high-GI options, will provide the best variety and feelings of psychological well-being. The occasional mini chocolate bar may not be the best high-GI fuel during exercise from a scientific point of view, but in the final stages of the Ironman, it may boost your morale enough to keep you going. These psychological factors cannot be underestimated.

11

RECOVERY: THE CASE FOR HIGH-GI FOODS

*A*FTER EXERCISE, YOUR muscles are hungry for carbohydrate. If you postpone consuming carbohydrate after exercise, you'll delay muscle-glycogen replenishment and could become fatigued.

- If you're a recreational exerciser, an adequate carbohydrate intake over the next few days will ensure that your muscles are ready for another session.
- If you're participating in strenuous training, particularly when two or more training sessions are part of your daily routine, rapid glycogen replenishment is vital. Eat or drink carbohydrate within 30 minutes of strenuous exercise when you plan to train again within a few hours. On consecutive days of competition, this recovery strategy will also assist in restocking your glycogen stores for the next event.

RECOVERY AFTER EXERCISE

In the immediate post-exercise period, high-GI carbohydrates are best because they are digested and
absorbed much faster and stimulate more insulin—the
hormone responsible for getting glucose into the muscle
and storing it as glycogen. Most athletes prefer high-
carbohydrate drinks because they are usually thirsty
rather than hungry after strenuous exercise. A drink also
aids rehydration.

Sports or electrolyte-replacement drinks are ideal for
replacing fluids and providing an immediate and convenient source of high-GI carbohydrate.

After this initial "dose" of recovery carbs, try to make
sure your next meal or snack (within two hours) includes
intermediate- to high-GI foods.

RECOVERY FORMULA

The amount of carbohydrate required to kick off the
recovery process is about 1.5 grams per kilogram of
body weight. Most people need between 50 and approximately 100 grams of carbohydrate in the immediate
post-exercise period. The table on page 55 outlines a list
of convenient high-GI foods and sports drinks suitable
for recovery.

■

**Postponing carbohydrate consumption after exercise delays
muscle-glycogen replenishment and can cause fatigue.**

■

Serving Sizes of High-GI Foods to Enhance Recovery

FOOD	GI VALUE	SERVING SIZE = 50 GRAMS CARBOHYDRATE	SERVING SIZE = 100 GRAMS CARBOHYDRATE
White or brown bread	70	3 slices (3 oz.)	6 slices (6 oz.)
Kellogg's Rice Krispies™	82	2¼ cups (2 oz. + 6 oz. milk)	4½ cups (4 oz. + 12 oz. milk)
Kellogg's Corn Flakes™	92	1½ cups (1½ oz. + 6 oz. milk)	3 cups (3 oz. + 12 oz. milk)
Watermelon	72	4⅓ cups (1¼ lbs.)	8⅔ cups (2½ lbs.)
Honey graham crackers	74	9 squares (2¼ oz.)	18 squares (4½ oz.)
Rice cakes	78	7 rice cakes (2½ oz.)	14 rice cakes (5 oz.)
English muffins, toasted	77	2 whole muffins (4 oz.)	4 whole muffins (8 oz.)
Instant rice, cooked	74	1⅓ cups (7 oz.)	2⅔ cups (14 oz.)
Jelly beans	78	20 large (2 oz.)	40 large (4 oz.)
Gatorade™	89	3½ cups (28 oz.)	7 cups (56 oz.)

Females weighing about 110 pounds should aim to eat 75 grams of carbohydrate.

Males weighing about 165 pounds should aim to eat 112 grams of carbohydrate.

■

Better fueling—not more training —can give you the competitive edge!

▪

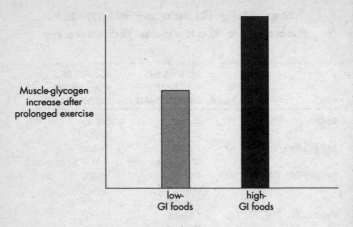

Figure 6. Comparison of the effect of low- and high-GI foods on replenishment of muscle-glycogen levels after exercise.

◀ 12 ▶

THE IMPORTANCE OF WEIGHT CONTROL

A HIGH-CARBOHYDRATE, low-GI diet can help you manage your weight and body-fat levels with greater ease. Low-GI foods help you fill up more easily, which is useful if you need to control your food intake to stay lean or reduce to a certain weight for competition.

The good news is that carbohydrate foods are filling, not fattening. Fatty foods, in particular, have only a weak effect on satisfying our appetites relative to the number of calories they provide. Carbohydrate foods make you feel fuller than fats and don't end up on your body in places where you least want them!

In Australian studies, people were given a range of individual foods that contained equal numbers of calories, after which their satiety (fullness) responses were compared. Researchers found that the most filling foods were those that contained fewer calories per gram (were the least "energy-dense"). These foods included oatmeal, apples, oranges, and pasta. Eating more of these foods satisfies your appetite without providing excess calories. On the other hand, foods that provide a lot of calories per gram, such as croissants, chocolate, and peanuts, were the least satisfying. These foods are more likely to leave us wanting more, leading to what scientists call "passive over-consumption," or overeating without even realizing it.

After energy density (number of calories), the researchers found that the second-best predictor of satiety was a food's GI value—the lower the GI value, the more the food satisfied hunger. Indeed, there are now over 17 studies that confirm low-GI foods suppress hunger longer than high-GI foods.

There are probably several mechanisms responsible for this, including:

- Low-GI foods remain longer in the small intestine, triggering receptors that tell the brain there's still food in the gut to be digested.
- High-GI foods may stimulate hunger because they cause blood-glucose levels to rapidly rise, and then fall.
- Stress hormones such as adrenaline and cortisol are released when glucose levels rebound after eating high-GI foods. Both hormones tend to stimulate appetite.
- Low-GI foods may be more filling simply because they are often less energy-dense than their high GI counterparts. The naturally high fiber content of many low-GI foods increases their bulk without increasing their calorie content.

What's more, even when the calorie intake is the same, people eating low-GI foods may lose more weight than those eating high-GI foods. In a South African study, investigators divided overweight volunteers into two groups: one group ate high-GI foods, the other ate low-GI foods. The amount of calories, fat, protein, carbohydrate, and fiber in the diet was the same for both groups; only the GI values of the diets were different. The low-GI group included foods such as lentils and oatmeal in their diet and excluded high-GI foods such as potatoes and white bread. After 12 weeks, the volunteers in the group eating low-GI foods had lost, on average, nearly 20 pounds—more than 4 pounds more than people in the group eating the diet of high-GI foods.

How did the low-GI diet work? The most significant finding was the different effects of the two diets on the level of insulin in the blood. Low-GI foods resulted in lower levels of insulin circulating in the bloodstream. Insulin plays a key role because this hormone is not only involved in regulating blood-sugar levels, it also helps to determine when and how we store fat. High levels of insulin often exist in obese people, in those with high blood-fat levels (either cholesterol or triglyceride), and in those with heart disease. This study suggested that the low insulin responses associated with low-GI foods helped the body burn more fat rather than store it.

There are other reasons why low-GI diets might aid weight loss, too: when people first begin a diet, their metabolic rate drops in response to the reduction in food intake. One study, however, found that the metabolic rate had dropped less after one week on a low-GI diet than on a conventional high-carbohydrate diet. The same study suggested that the low-GI diet helped to preserve lean body mass better, which could explain the higher metabolic rate.

FACTORS THAT INFLUENCE BODY WEIGHT

Like most health conditions, there are many different causes for obesity, some of which include our genetic makeup, hormone levels, environmental factors, psychological issues, and metabolic considerations.

For most of us, even without much conscious effort, our bodies maintain a relatively constant weight, often despite huge variations in how much we eat. For a proportion of people who are overweight, this apparent balancing of energy intake and output seems lost or inoperative. So, despite every fad diet, every exercise program, even operations and medications, body weight can steadily increase over the years, regardless of all efforts to control it.

It has always been said that our weight is a result of how much we consume in relation to how much we burn up. So, if we take in too much (overeat) and don't burn up enough (don't exercise), we are likely to put on weight.

The question is: how much, of what, is too much?

The answer is not a simple one: not all foods that we eat are equal and no two bodies are the same, given the wide variety of special factors we've outlined above.

WHAT'S INVOLVED?

As we mentioned earlier, people are overweight for many different reasons. Some people believe they gain weight just from looking at food, while others say they have only to walk past a bakery to pack on a few extra pounds. Still other folks blame themselves because they eat too much. It is clear that a combination of social, genetic, dietary, metabolic, psychological (and emotional) factors combine to influence our weight.

YOUR FAMILY TREE

Research shows that a child born to overweight parents is much more likely to be overweight than one whose parents were not overweight. It may sound like an excuse, but studies in twins provide evidence that our body weight and shape are at least partially determined by our genes.

Identical twins tend to be similar in body weight even if they are raised apart. Even twins adopted as infants show the body-fat profile of their true parents rather than that of their adoptive parents. These findings suggest that our genes are a stronger determinant of weight than our environment, which includes the food we eat.

How do genes play a role? It seems that information stored in our genes governs our tendency to store calories as either fat or as lean muscle tissue. Overfeeding a large group of identical twins confirmed that within each pair, weight gain was similar. The amount of weight gained between sets of identical twins varied greatly, however. From this, researchers concluded that our genes control the way our bodies respond to overeating. Some sets of twins gained a lot of weight, while others gained only a little, even though all were consuming an equivalent amount of excess calories.

It's Not Just Genetics

DESPITE A GENETIC PREDISPOSITION, you can only gain weight if you take in more energy than you use. We know that obesity has many causes—for example, eating too much, exercising too little, genetics, aging, eating a high-fat diet—all play a part. But what it all boils down to is that if we take in too much (overeat) and don't burn up enough (don't exercise) we are likely to put on weight.

All this isn't to say that if your parents were overweight, you should resign yourself to being overweight. But it may help you understand why you have to watch your weight while other people seemingly don't have to watch theirs.

So, if you were born with a tendency to be overweight, why does it matter what you eat? The answer is that foods (or more correctly, nutrients) are not equal in their effects on body weight. In particular, the way the body responds to dietary fat makes matters worse.

Some scientists believe that fat is fattening because the body has a very limited ability to store protein and carbohydrate but a very large capacity to store fat. Our bodies burn protein and carbohydrate first, and preferentially store dietary fat. Every day we will burn virtually all the carbohydrate and protein we ingest. In a steady state of weight balance, though, the amount of fat we burn each day must equal the amount we eat. (If we eat a high-fat diet, then our body fat stores must expand so that the level of free fatty acids in the blood is high enough to correspond to what we're eating. That's why a high-fat diet brings about a high-fat body.)

Counting the Calories in Our Nutrients

ALL FOODS CONTAIN calories. Often the caloric content of a food is considered a measure of how fattening it is. Of all the nutrients in food that we consume, carbohydrate and protein yields the fewest calories per gram.

carbohydrate	4 calories per gram
protein	4 calories per gram
alcohol	7 calories per gram
fat	9 calories per gram

While you may not have been born owning the best set of genes for the current environment, you can still influence your weight by the lifestyle choices you make. The message is simply this: if you believe that you are at risk of being overweight, you should think seriously about minimizing fat and eating more carbohydrate.

HOW FAST YOUR MOTOR RUNS

Our genetic makeup also underlies our metabolism, which is basically how many calories we burn per minute. Bodies, like cars, differ in this regard. A V-8 consumes more fuel to run than a small four-cylinder car. A bigger body usually requires more calories than a smaller one.

Everyone has a resting metabolic rate, which is a measure of the amount of calories our bodies use when we are at rest. When a car is stationary, the engine idles—using just enough fuel to keep the motor running. When we are asleep, our engine keeps running, too (for example, our heart keeps beating) and we use a minimum number of calories. This is our basal metabolic rate.

When we start exercising, or even just moving around, the number of calories, or the amount of fuel we use, increases. However, the largest amount (around 70 percent) of the calories used in a 24-hour period are those used to maintain our basic body functioning.

Since our resting metabolic rate is where most of the calories we eat are used, it is a significant determinant of our body weight. The lower your resting energy expenditure, the greater your risk of gaining weight, and vice versa.

◀ 13 ▶

CASE STUDY #1:
JIM

$\mathcal{J}$IM IS AN 18-year-old college football player who recently moved from a small rural town to join one of the best college teams in the country. Playing college (and eventually professional) football is Jim's dream. Wanting to make a big impression during his first few weeks at training, Jim gave his all. At first he felt fine, but after one week of training twice almost every day he felt exhausted, and was frankly "off the pace." Sensing that Jim was struggling, the coach took him aside and recommended he speak to a registered dietitian about his diet and recovery strategies.

Jim's Weekly Training Program

Morning weight/circuit training: 2 or 3 sessions per
week of 1 to 1½ hours

Afternoon football/fitness sessions: 4 sessions of 2
to 2½ hours per week

CONSULTATION WITH THE SPORTS DIETITIAN

Jim was a bit wary of changing his diet; he wondered
how eating differently could help him on the football
field. The dietitian explained that carbohydrates were
the key to energy and recovery. His diet at the moment
was far too low in carbohydrate to get him through the
tough pre-season training. The dietitian also explained
that eating carbohydrate regularly was important, and
fueling up immediately (within 30 minutes) after training sessions helped to replace the body's carbohydrate
stores more quickly. Timing was important because
between morning and afternoon training, his body had
less than six hours to refuel. More rapidly absorbing
carbs, or those with intermediate to high GI values, were
also better for refueling as they replenished the body's
carbohydrate or glycogen levels faster.

The dietitian also explained that to help Jim maintain
his body weight and stay lean he should:

- eat lean meats or cut off the fat
- remove skin from chicken

▶ eat reduced-fat dairy products
▶ minimize use of oils, butter, or margarine

HIGH-GI FUEL TO THE RESCUE

Jim noticed the other players were already using foods and sports drinks to their advantage. They consumed sports drinks with glucose (high GI value) to begin the refueling and rehydration process right after training and chose intermediate- to high-GI breads, cereals, or fruit to boost their recovery (French bread, Cheerios, Corn Chex, granola bars, pineapple, or watermelon). These foods were available at training so he could start the refueling process before going home.

The dietitian also organized cooking classes to give him the confidence to prepare different carbohydrate-based meals for himself. But Jim now knew that when recovery time was short, higher-GI carbohydrates were best.

RESULTS

Jim noticed the difference in his performance after being on the high-carbohydrate diet for only a few days. He felt fresher at afternoon training and could really power through the sprint sessions, which had been like torture before. Including more carbohydrate in his diet and refueling with higher-GI carbohydrates really helped him. He knew he still had a lot of work to do before the competition season kicked off, but with the right fuel, a great attitude, and some raw talent, he knew he was ready for some of his best-ever performances.

Meal Plan for Jim

Aim: To provide sufficient carbohydrate and energy and to assist recovery rate by incorporating high-GI liquids and intermediate- to high-GI meals after training.

	NOTES ON GI

8:30 A.M. Immediately post training
1 quart sports/electrolyte drink (Gatorade™)

	Post Training Intermediate- to high- GI choices
9:00 A.M. Breakfast	
1 piece of fruit	Pineapple, watermelon
2 cups of cereal	Puffed wheat, corn flakes,
2 cups of 2% milk	raisin bran
2 slices white or whole-wheat toast	White or whole wheat kaiser
(no butter) with 1 tablespoon honey	roll or French bread
1 glass of fruit juice (8 oz.)	Pineapple

11:30 A.M. Snack
1 sandwich with 3 oz.
  lean meat filling (turkey breast,
  lean roast beef)
1 piece of fruit (any type)
1 non-fat yogurt (8 oz.)

1:00 P.M. Lunch
3 slices rye bread filled with 3 oz.
  boiled ham and 2 oz. American
  cheese or any of the following: lean
  meat, chicken, reduced-fat cheese,
  egg, canned tuna in spring water or
  canned salmon
2 pieces of fresh fruit (any type)

1 pint (16 oz.) of low-fat, flavored milk

2:30 P.M. Snack
Fruit smoothie or a liquid meal
(such as Ensure Light or Super Shake)

**3:30–5:30 P.M. Pre- and
during training**
2 quarts of sports/electrolyte drink   High-GI drink Gatorade™ (78)

5:30 P.M. After training
1 quart sports/electrolyte drink or
  carb loader   High-GI drink for recovery

7:00 P.M. Dinner
Serving of lean meat (5 oz.),
  or skinless chicken (6 oz.), or
  fish (8 oz.)—grilled or cooked
  with minimum oil
Large serving of rice (1⅓ cups)   High-GI rice on training
  or pasta (3 cups) or 2 medium   nights, pasta most others
  potatoes

1 cup serving of vegetables or large
  tossed green salad (no-oil dressing)
4 slices of white bread or 2 rolls   High-GI French bread
  (no butter)   on training nights

9:00 P.M. Snack
2 pieces of fresh fruit in a smoothie
  or fruit and yogurt

Dietary Analysis:

Energy: 4,458 calories   **Fat:** 74 g (15%)
Protein: 189 g (17%)   **Carbohydrate:** 759 g (68%)

14

CASE STUDY #2:
ANALISE

ANALISE, A 16-YEAR-OLD full-time ballet student, had a dream: to be a dancer with a major ballet company. When she started to mature at 13, she found she could no longer eat anything as she used to. Extra weight started to pile on. First she tried all the diets given to her by the other ballet students, but she always felt hungry and craved chocolate. Getting nowhere by herself, her mother took her to see a sports dietitian.

CONSULTATION WITH THE
SPORTS DIETITIAN

At their first meeting the dietitian took a history of Analise's weight and eating patterns and found that a typical day's meals for Analise included:

- A slice of white toast with butter and a cup of strong black tea for breakfast
- Two crispbreads with butter and a cup of black tea for a morning snack
- A green salad, an apple, and a cup of black tea for lunch
- A chocolate bar and a can of diet cola during the afternoon (waiting at the train station)
- Steamed veggies, sometimes steamed chicken, and a cup of black tea for dinner
- A chocolate bar or chocolate cookies and tea for an evening snack

The dietitian explained that this diet was high in fat and too low in protein, carbohydrate, calcium, and iron. She explained that:

- Gaining a little body weight and fat is part of the maturation process and that the best way to control body fat was with a sensible diet, not starving.
- Cravings are to be expected when you're hungry. After working hard in class all day with virtually no food, chocolate is just too tempting. Eating more carbohydrate on a regular basis would help Analise control her chocolate cravings.
- Analise needed a dietary strategy to give her sufficient fuel to get through the day without feeling hungry. Carbohydrates (especially low-GI carbs) would help her to feel fuller, give her more energy, and provide less fat than other foods she'd been eating.

Analise's meal plan, based on reducing fat intake and boosting carbohydrate, meant eating more pasta, rice, bread, fruit, and vegetables and less high-fat food such as butter and chocolate. Chocolate was not totally out of the question, but she had to cut back to get her body-fat levels going in the right direction. The dietitian also explained that reducing the cups of tea would help Analise maintain adequate iron levels, because the tannin in tea reduces iron absorption.

Analise had some questions about the meal plan.

Could she really lose weight eating this much?

The dietitian explained that the size or appearance of foods is often deceiving. Although some high-fat foods like chocolate look compact, and foods like bread and vegetables may take up more space on the plate, the fat and calorie values of high-fat foods are much greater than those of bread and vegetables. The fat figures in the back of this book were a real surprise to Analise. She was also surprised to learn that the fat we eat is converted into body fat faster and more easily than anything else we eat.

Should she cut out chocolate all together?

The dietitian explained that giving up chocolate is really not necessary and is almost impossible unless you live somewhere where there's no chocolate at all. Eating chocolate as a treat, not as a substitute meal, is the key.

How could she avoid feeling too full and having a bloated stomach during class?

Foods with a high fiber content (including many salad veggies) produce more gas in the intestine, which can cause bloating. The dietitian showed Analise how she could increase her intake of low-GI carbs throughout the day without feeling bloated.

RESULTS

At first Analise kept thinking that she was eating too much. But she was able to avoid the chocolate vending machine on the station platform on the way home because she felt fuller during the day. The really high-carb, low-GI foods reduced her hunger. Her body-fat level (measured with body-fat or skinfold calipers) dropped steadily each week. She thought it almost unbelievable to be able to drop fat without starving! An added bonus was her improved energy levels and concentration in class, not to mention her mood, which was more relaxed and cheerful.

Analise's Meal Plan

Aim: To provide a regular supply of carbohydrate, with less fat. GI values should be intermediate to low to assist with satiety.

NOTES ON GI	
8:00 A.M. Breakfast	**Intermediate to low GI**
1 piece of fruit	Fresh apple, grapefruit, kiwi
½–⅔ cup bran cereal	All Bran™, oats, Raisin Bran™
4 oz. skim milk	
1 slice whole-grain toast (no butter) and 1 teaspoon spreadable fruit	Oat, barley, or mixed-grain breads
1 cup decaffeinated coffee	
10:30 A.M. Snack	
Non-fat fruit yogurt with artificial sweetener	
1:00 P.M. Lunch	
1 sandwich—protein options include: 2 oz. of chicken, turkey, canned tuna in water, salmon, reduced-fat cheese, lean ham, or roast meat	Oat, barley, or heavy-grain bread
2 cups of salad with 2 tablespoons light dressing	
1 piece of fruit	Peach, pear, or plum
Water or decaf diet beverage	
3:30 P.M. Snack	
1 raisin toast or ½ English muffin with 1 teaspoon jam	Raisin bread or grain muffin
7:00 P.M. Dinner	**Intermediate to low GI**
3 oz. serving of lean meat, or 4 oz. skinless chicken or 5 oz. grilled fish, all cooked in minimum or no oil	
1 medium potato or 1 cup pasta or ⅔ cup rice	New boiled potatoes, pasta or Basmati or brown rice

7:00 P.M. Dinner
1 cup serving of vegetables or salad
   with 2 tablespoons light dressing
Water or decaf diet beverage

9:30 P.M. Snack
1 8 oz. glass of skim milk
1 slice raisin toast with 1 teaspoon
   spreadable fruit

Dietary Analysis:

Energy: 1,305 calories

Fat: 20 g (14%)

Calcium: 1,225 mg (daily calcium requirement for 16-year-old female is 1,200-1,500 mg)

Protein: 78 g (24%)

Carbohydrate: 215 g (66%)

Iron: 14–18 mg (above the recommended daily intake)

◀ 15 ▶

CASE STUDY #3:
IAN

*I*AN IS A **26**-YEAR-OLD physical education teacher
and enthusiastic triathlete. He has competed in the
Olympic distance for the past five years but is now trying to qualify for the Ironman triathlon in Hawaii. Ian
wanted everything to be just right for his first Ironman
race so he could qualify. He approached a sports dietitian to help him plan his dietary strategy and brought a
list of questions to ask.

HOW MUCH CARBOHYDRATE
DOES HE NEED IN HIS TRAINING DIET?

The approximate amount of carbohydrate Ian needs is
calculated by multiplying his weight by the carbohydrate
requirement appropriate for his activity level.

Ian's weight:	165 lbs. (75 kg)
Approximate carbohydrate requirement for his activity level (see page 34):	8 g/kg
Daily carbohydrate needs for training:	75 x 8 = 600 g

This amount of carbohydrate may be too difficult to achieve with food. Liquid carbohydrate supplements (such as sports drinks) can help boost carbohydrate intake.

Ian's Training Program

	A.M. TRAINING	P.M. TRAINING
Monday	1.8-mile swim	Track session + 4-mile run
Tuesday	1.8-mile swim	60-mile cycle
Wednesday	Rest	9-mile run
Thursday	1.8-mile swim	60-mile cycle
Friday	1.8-mile swim	30-mile easy cycle
Saturday	93-mile cycle	1.8-mile swim
Sunday	Rest	18-mile run

IAN'S VITAL STATISTICS

Height: 5'8" (70 inches)

Weight: 165 lbs. (has lost 9 lbs. over the past 3 months)

Sum of 8 skinfolds: 50 mm (indicates that Ian is very lean)

HOW CAN HE INCORPORATE THE GLYCEMIC INDEX INTO HIS TRAINING DIET?

Ian can incorporate the glycemic index into his diet mainly by including high-GI drinks (such as sports drinks) during and after training. Intermediate- to high-GI foods after training also help to speed up recovery. At other times, it's more important to eat sufficient carbohydrate—whatever the GI value. Most athletes requiring the amount of carbohydrate that Ian does will feel more comfortable with moderate- to lower-fiber carbohydrate choices (such as white bread, rice, and pasta instead of the whole-grain varieties, for example). Otherwise the sheer volume of the carbohydrate and fiber becomes too bulky and bloating.

WHY HAS HE BEEN SO FATIGUED LATELY?

Fatigue is a generalized symptom that has numerous causes. Dietary factors that should be considered include:

- **Low iron intake.** If your iron levels are low, then increased amounts of high-iron foods need to be included in your diet. Iron deficiency occurs even in athletes with adequate iron intake, and is more common in endurance athletes.
- **Inadequate carbohydrate intake.** It's possible to feel fatigued if your muscle-glycogen stores are low, which suggests that you're consuming inadequate amounts of carbohydrate throughout the day. Tiredness can also be due to low blood sugar, which can happen if there's a long period

between meals. Low blood sugar (hypoglycemia) commonly occurs in early morning or afternoon training sessions when you consume insufficient amounts of carbohydrate before the session.

- **Overtraining.** Having too many strenuous workouts is a common problem with endurance athletes. Training programs need to be tailored to the individual, incorporating their personal needs for sleep and taking into account their occupational demands.

- **Viral illness.** A number of medical conditions— not just viruses—are potential causes of fatigue. Ian would benefit from a referral to a sports physician and an exercise physiologist to help determine which factors in particular are causing his fatigue.

DOES HE NEED TO GLYCOGEN-LOAD PRIOR TO THE EVENT?

Since the event will be longer than 2 hours (about 11 hours actually), yes! The meal plan outlined below shows how he can glycogen-load using the modified regimen. This regimen involves tapered training and a high-carbohydrate diet three to four days prior to the race. The diet should provide about 9 to 10 grams of carbohydrate per kilogram of body weight. Check the meal plan for guidance.

WHAT WOULD BE THE BEST PRE-EVENT MEAL?

Ian would benefit from trying a low-GI meal in practice to see how this worked for him. To maintain gastric comfort, the best low-GI options would include lower-fiber choices such as white pasta, rolled oats, or a liquid low-fat meal (Ensure Light or Super Shake, for example).

HOW CAN HE MAINTAIN ENERGY THROUGHOUT THE EVENT?

During the event, maintaining energy and hydration will be a major factor influencing his performance. Sports drinks would be the best option to replace energy and fluids during the race. Because sports drinks have a high GI value they will be a rapidly absorbed and easily available source of carbohydrate. Other high-GI options include carbohydrate gels, jelly beans, or honey sandwiches on high-GI (white French) bread. Because Ian will only be able to carry a small amount of the high-GI food options, the sports drink will probably provide the basis of his refueling strategy, with foods offering minor support.

To prevent boredom and boost morale, some of the other offerings at the aid stations (chocolate chip cookies, sandwiches, colas) could be included in smaller quantities as treats. These provide more of a psychological incentive than physiological boost. Although a little caffeine in the cola drink may help with fatigue later in the race due to its stimulant properties, Ian needs to limit caffeine ingestion to avoid dehydration problems (because it takes longer to empty from the stomach, caffeine can compromise hydration). Caffeine may also be subject to drug testing.

Ian's Meal Plan

Aim: To provide sufficient carbohydrate and nutrition for peak performance. The meal plan should include intermediate- to high-GI meals or snacks after training sessions to help maximize the rate of glycogen replacement.

	NOTES ON GI	
Regular training	**Post-training intermediate to high GI choices**	**Loading phase**
Breakfast		
1–2 pieces of fresh fruit	Pineapple, watermelon	Same breakfast
2 cups General Mills Honey Nut Cheerios™ cereal	Kellogg's Rice Krispies™, Quaker Puffed Wheat™, General Mills Total™	
1 cup (8 oz.) 2% milk		
3 slices of toast with 1 tablespoon honey (no butter)	Kaiser roll or French bread	
16 oz. orange juice		
Snack		
1 banana and 2 oatmeal raisin cookies (2 oz.) 8 oz. glass of juice (any type)		Same as training plan but add in an additional banana or a low-fat fruit muffin
Lunch		
3 slices rye bread (made with 6 oz. of cheese, chicken, lean meat, egg, tuna, or salmon) 1 piece fruit 8 oz. Gatorade™		Same lunch but add in ½ jelly sandwich for extra carbohydrate

REGULAR TRAINING	POST-TRAINING INTERMEDIATE TO HIGH GI CHOICES	LOADING PHASE
Snack		
Fruit smoothie made with 8 oz. 2% milk		Use a liquid meal (such as Ensure Light or Super Shake) or carb loader.
Before and during training: Sports drink (volume dependent on session type and duration)— at least 1 quart		Be sure to replace fluids
Dinner		
Medium serving of lean meat or skinless chicken (5 oz.), or fish (6–8 oz.) or a vegetarian meal		Same dinner
Large serving of potato, rice or pasta (1½–2 cups)	High-GI rice (such as cooked instant rice); great after hard afternoon training sessions	
Medium serving of vegetables or tossed green salad (at least 1 cup) with fat-free dressing		
4 slices of bread or two rolls	High-GI bread (kaiser roll, French bread)	
2 pieces of fresh fruit	Pineapple, watermelon	
1 glass any juice (8 oz.)		
Snack		
4 pieces raisin toast with jelly or honey		Add in a carb-loader drink or a liquid meal (such as Ensure Light or Super Shake)
1 glass fruit juice		

Dietary Analysis (Training):

Energy: 4,214 calories   **Protein:** 168 g (16%)
Fat: 86 g (18%)   **Carbohydrate:** 692 g (66%)

Dietary Analysis (Loading):

Energy: 4,531 calories   **Fat:** 88 g (17%)
Protein: 171 g (15%)   **Carbohydrate:** 767 g (68%)

THE PRE-EVENT MEAL PLAN FOR IAN

This meal should be consumed about two to three hours prior to competition. Ian had tried out the low-GI meal in training and wanted to use it in competition. The meals he found most comfortable included:

- Liquid meal (Ensure Light   GI = 39
  or Super Shake) plus a serving
  of stewed apple
- Rolled oats with skim milk   GI = 44
  and orange juice
- Lentil soup and grapes   GI = 47

RESULTS

Ian went on to qualify for Hawaii. Being prepared for this race was crucial to his best performance. Ian described the Hawaii Ironman as "awesome"—one of the best experiences of his life—and it was made more enjoyable by being well prepared and well fueled.

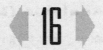

16

CASE STUDY #4:
JOHN

*J*OHN IS A SINGLE man. He works as a full-time fire-fighter and takes college courses at night. As an athlete, John competes in bi- and triathlons. He wants to lose 12 pounds, and believes his physical stamina and athletic performance will improve at an optimal weight of 175 pounds.

John's Training Program

Runs: 4 to 6 times a week for 40 minutes (3 miles)
Bikes: 3 times a week for 90 minutes
Weight trains: 5 to 7 times a week for 30 minutes

JOHN'S VITAL STATISTICS
   Age: 25
   Height: 5'9"

continued

Weight: 187 pounds (Although muscular, John is still at 110 percent of reasonable body weight for height and body frame. He has gained 12 pounds in the past 9 years.)

Goal weight: 170 pounds

JOHN'S "BEFORE" DIET:

Breakfast: Two to three cups Rice Chex, 16 oz. 2% milk

Snack: Banana, pear, 2 carrots

Lunch: Two slices white sandwich bread, 3 ozs. roast beef, 2 oz. pretzels, 1 cup strawberries, 32 ozs. Gatorade™

Dinner: Grilled steak (16 oz.), 1½ cups green beans with approximately 2 tablespoons butter, 2 cups linguine with approximately 1 cup cream sauce, 32 oz. Gatorade™

Late-night snack: Twenty saltines, 32 oz. Gatorade™

John's "Before" Nutritional Analysis:

Calories: 5,500

Carbohydrate: 554 g (41%)

Protein: 244 g (18%)

Fat: 252 g (41%)

GI value: 77

CONSULTATION WITH THE DIETITIAN

Even taking his extreme workout schedule into account, John is overconsuming calories by about 50 percent. Even in an athlete's body, this means weight gain (in the form of body fat). All of the macronutrients in his diet (carbohydrates, protein, and fat) need to be reduced to bring the calories down to a reasonable level. John needs to reduce his caloric intake to 2,800 calories, which will meet his basal metabolic requirements as well as his workout energy needs.

GI-SPECIFIC COUNSELING:

John is consuming a high-GI diet. In addition to reducing his caloric intake in the forms of protein foods (steak and roast beef, for example) and his condiments (such as butter and cream sauces), he will also need to reduce his carbohydrates.

By choosing low-GI cereals (such as Bran Buds, muesli, old-fashioned oatmeal) instead of high-GI types (including Rice Chex and corn flakes), and low-GI breads (such as whole-wheat pita, 100% whole-wheat, or whole-grain pumpernickel bread) instead of white sandwich bread, he would feel fuller for longer periods of time. His high-GI snacks could be replaced with light yogurt or low-fat milk, oatmeal or Social Tea biscuits and fruit. One 32-ounce bottle of Gatorade™ during and after a workout period would suffice on a daily basis as long as he consumed at least 80 ounces of water as well.

JOHN'S NEW, LOW-GI MENU:

Breakfast: Two cups Quaker Oats oat bran cereal, 12 oz. 1% milk, large apple, water

Snack: One cup grapes

Lunch: Two slices whole-grain pumpernickel, 3 oz. lean roast beef, 1 tablespoon mayonnaise, a sandwich bag of raw vegetables (baby carrots, celery, pepper strips, for example), large pear, 2 oatmeal cookies, water

Snack: Low-fat granola bar, 8 oz. 1% milk

Dinner: One and one-half cups long-grain rice, 6 oz. chicken rosemary, 2 cups steamed broccoli with 2 pats butter and 2 tablespoons slivered almonds, water

Snack: Small apple cinnamon muffin (from mix), 8 oz. 1% milk

John's "After" Nutritional Analysis:

Calories: 2,800   **Carbohydrate:** 379 g (54%)
Protein: 150 g (21%)   **Fat:** 77 g (25%)
GI value: 46

RESULTS

After just five weeks, John had dropped 7½ pounds, came in 66th out of more than 200 competitors in a biathlon and had shortened his mile by 40 seconds. He reached his goal weight of 170 pounds after 10 weeks. It's been four years since John has been incorporating low-GI foods into his meal/snack planning.

He is still an elite athlete, and maintains a healthy weight of 171 pounds. John tells us: "I never dreamed I could run so fast or bike so long on half the calories I was used to eating!"

◀ 17 ▶

YOUR QUESTIONS ANSWERED

What about the pre-event meal before high-intensity or non-endurance exercise?

As we mentioned earlier, there is some evidence that eating low-GI carbohydrates before endurance exercise may help enhance performance. Studies on shorter-term exercise have not yet been done, so we need to await further research. At this stage, there are many factors to consider when you're planning an optimal pre-event meal, including the timing, the fiber content (to prevent bloating), the fat content, and the GI value. Much of the advice about pre-event eating has come from practical experience, and surprisingly little from scientific research. Because you need to consider so many factors, the best advice for shorter-term exercise is to consider the list of optimal pre-event eating strategies and experiment with foods or meals to determine what works best for you.

If a person were to eat both protein and carbohydrates during training and before a race, how much of each should they eat?

For most people, a training diet should provide approximately 60 percent of calories from carbohydrate, 15 to 20 percent of calories from protein, and the rest from fat. To calculate the amount of carbohydrate that's best for you, turn to "What's Your Activity Level?" in chapter 7.

An athlete's protein needs generally range between 1.2 and 2 grams of protein per kilogram of body weight. Prior to competition, there's no specific need for additional protein. In fact, in most cases athletes require extra carbohydrate to ensure that liver glycogen and blood-sugar levels are optimal. By the way, scientists no longer recommend the glycogen-loading protocols of years past, which endorsed a low-carbohydrate, higher-protein diet to enhance loading. For more on this subject, see the box "Eat to Compete: Carbohydrate Loading" on page 42.

What should be the overall glycemic index value of an athlete's diet?

Good question! Unfortunately, scientists have yet to answer it. There is evidence that diets with higher GI values increase the glycogen storage in the muscle of sedentary individuals. This may help athletes to store glycogen more effectively on a day-to-day basis. A high GI value has been shown to enhance the rate of recovery of muscle glycogen after exercise. During exercise, food with high GI values is required to provide a rapidly available fuel source.

I am a recreational jogger; what should be the GI value of my overall diet?

If you exercise to lose weight, there may be some benefit in choosing low-GI carbohydrates at each meal for their high satiety value. Generally speaking, it's important for recreational joggers to have sufficient carbohydrate in their diet for good health and energy. Since the time to restore glycogen after a workout is likely to be longer than for elite athletes, there is less need to eat high-GI carbohydrates immediately after exercise.

What about eating between heats and trials over the day?

There is insufficient scientific evidence to recommend a particular GI value between events at present. However, it makes sense to include carbohydrates that are rapidly absorbed (higher-GI foods) on a regular basis over the day. Eat little and often. Maintain fluid intake to optimize hydration. During shorter (less than one hour) breaks, drinking rapidly absorbed liquids is probably best. For longer breaks, we recommend eating small low-fat, high-carb snacks (including rice cakes, soft fruits, honey sandwiches, sports bars, and so on).

Is there an easy way to tell if a food has a high or low GI value?

No. The only way to tell is to measure the blood-sugar response to that food. Generally, foods that break down quickly during digestion have the highest GI values. GI values cannot be predicted from the chemical composition of the food or the GI value of related foods. Milling and grinding break down the cellular structure of grains and tend to speed up the rate of digestion, which increases the GI value. Cooking increases the digestibility of starch, and may also increase the GI value. It might seem surprising, but removing the dietary fiber in bread, rice, or pasta has little effect on GI values. However, the viscous fiber found in fruits and some grains (such as oats and barley) may account for their lower GI values. In some instances, fat slows the digestion process and lowers the GI value.

◀ 18 ▶

LET'S TALK GLYCEMIC LOAD

*I*N ADDITION TO the GI values we provide in this book, our tables also include the glycemic load (GL) value for average-sized food portions. Taken together, the glycemic index and glycemic load provide you with all the information you need to choose a diet brimming with health-boosting foods.

GLYCEMIC LOAD 101

A food's glycemic load results from the GI value and carbohydrate per serving of food. When we eat a carbohydrate-containing meal, our blood glucose first rises, then falls. The extent to which it rises and remains high is critically important to our health and depends on two things: the *amount* of a carbohydrate in the meal and the *nature* (GI value) of that carbohydrate. Both factors equally determine blood-glucose changes.

Researchers at Harvard University came up with a way of combining and describing these two factors with the term "glycemic load," which provides not only a measure of the level of glucose in the blood, but also the insulin demand produced by a normal serving of the food. Researchers measure GI values for fixed portions of foods containing a certain amount of carbohydrate (usually 50 grams). Then, as people eat different-sized portions of the same foods, we can work out the extent to which a certain portion of food will raise the blood-glucose level by calculating a glycemic load value for that amount of food.

To calculate glycemic load, multiply a food's GI value by the amount of carbohydrate in a particular serving size, then divide by 100.

■

Glycemic load = (GI value x carbohydrate per serving) ÷ 100

■

For example, a small apple has a GI value of 40 and contains 15 grams of carbohydrate. Its glycemic load is $(40 \times 15) \div 100 = 6$. A small 5-ounce potato has a GI value of 90 and 15 grams of carbohydrate. It has a glycemic load of $(90 \times 15) \div 100 = 14$. This means one small potato will raise your blood-glucose level higher than one apple.

■

Low GL = 10 or less
Intermediate GL = 11–19
High GL = 20 or more

■

How GI Values Affect Glycemic Load

THE GLYCEMIC LOAD is greatest for those foods that provide the highest-GI carbohydrate, particularly those we tend to eat in large quantities. Compare the glycemic load of the following foods to see how the serving size, as well as the GI value, help to determine the glycemic response:

Rice, 1 cup
Carbohydrates: 43
GI: 83
GL: 36
(83 × 43) ÷ 100 = 36

Spaghetti, 1 cup
Carbohydrates: 40
GI: 44
GL: 18
(44 × 40) ÷ 100 = 18

Some nutritionists argue that the glycemic load is an improvement on the glycemic index because it provides an estimate of both quantity *and* quality of carbohydrate (the GI value gives us just quality) in a diet. In large Harvard studies, however, researchers were able to predict disease risk from people's overall diet, as well as its glycemic load. Using the glycemic load strengthened the relationship, suggesting that the more frequently we consume high-carbohydrate, high-GI foods, the worse it is for our health. Carbohydrate by itself has no effect—in other words, there was no benefit to low carbohydrate intake over high carbohydrate intake, or vice versa.

Remember that the GL values we provide are for the standardized (nominal) portion sizes listed. If you eat a different portion size, then you'll need to calculate another GI value. Here's how: first, determine the size of your portion, then work out the available carbohydrate content of this weight (this value is listed next to the GL), then multiply by the food's GI value. For example, the nominal serving size listed for bran flakes is ½ cup, the available carbohydrate is 18 grams, and the GI value is 74. So the GL for a ½-cup serving of bran flakes is (74 × 18) ÷ 100 = 13. If, however, you normally eat 1 cup of bran flakes, you'd need to double the available carbohydrate (18 × 2 = 36), and the GL for your larger cereal portion would be (74 × 36) ÷ 100 = 27. These numbers show that the larger portion of cereal releases a larger quantity of glucose into the bloodstream.

We urge you not to make the mistake of using the glycemic load alone. If you do, you might find yourself eating a diet with very little carbohydrate but a lot of fat—especially saturated fat—and excessive amounts of protein. For your overall health, the fat, fiber, and micronutrient content of your diet is also important. A dietitian can guide you further with healthy food choices.

◀ 19 ▶

A TO Z
GI VALUES

$\mathcal{T}$HE TABLE IN this section will help you find a food's glycemic index value quickly and easily, because we've listed the foods alphabetically.

The list provides not only the food's GI value but also its glycemic load (GL = (carbohydrate content × GI value) ÷ 100). We calculate the glycemic load using a "nominal" serving size as well as the carbohydrate content of that serving—both of which we've also listed. That way, you can choose foods with either a low GI value or a low glycemic load. If your favorite food is both high-GI and high-GL, you can either cut down the serving size or dilute the GL by combining it with very-low-GI foods, such as rice and lentils.

For the first time, we've also included foods that have very little carbohydrate; their GI value is zero, indicated by [0]. Many vegetables, such as avocados and broccoli, and protein foods such as chicken, cheese, and tuna, fall into the low- or no-carbohydrate category. Most alcoholic beverages are also low in carbohydrate.

Key to the Table

GI Value: The glycemic index value for the food, where glucose equals 100

Nominal Serving Size: The portion of food tested

Net Carb per Serving: The total grams of carbs available to the body for digestion from the particular food in the specific serving size (total grams of carbs minus grams of fiber)

GL per Serving: Glycemic load of the food; this relates to the quantity of carbs that will enter the bloodstream for the particular food in the specific serving size

---

FOOD	GI Value	Nominal Serving Size	Net Carb per Serving	GL per Serving
A				
All-Bran®, breakfast cereal	30	½ cup	15	4
Almonds	[0]	1.75 oz	0	0
Angel food cake, 1 slice	67	¹⁄₁₂ cake	29	19
Apple, dried	29	9 rings	34	10
Apple, fresh, medium	38	4 oz	15	6
Apple juice, pure, unsweetened, reconstituted	40	8 oz	29	12
Apple muffin, small	44	3.5 oz	41	18
Apricots, canned in light syrup	64	4 halves	19	12
Apricots, dried	30	17 halves	27	8
Apricots, fresh, 3 medium	57	4 oz	9	5
Arborio, risotto rice, cooked	69	¾ cup	53	36
Artichokes (Jerusalem)	[0]	½ cup	0	0
Avocado	[0]	¼	0	0
B				
Bagel, white	72	½	35	25
Baked beans	38	⅔ cup	31	12
Baked beans, canned in tomato sauce	48	⅔ cup	15	7
Banana cake, 1 slice	47	⅛ cake	38	18
Banana, fresh, medium	52	4 oz	24	12
Barley, pearled, cooked	25	1 cup	42	11
Basmati rice, white, cooked	58	1 cup	38	22
Beef	[0]	4 oz	0	0
Beer	[0]	8 oz	10	0
Beets, canned	64	½ cup	7	5
Bengal gram dahl, chickpea	11	5 oz	36	4
Black bean soup	64	1 cup	27	17
Black beans, cooked	30	⅘ cup	23	7
Black-eyed peas, canned	42	⅔ cup	17	7

[0] indicates that the food has so little carbohydrate that the GI value cannot be tested. The GL, therefore, is 0.

FOOD	GI Value	Nominal Serving Size	Net Carb per Serving	GL per Serving
Blueberry muffin, small	59	3.5 oz	47	28
Bok choy, raw	[0]	1 cup	0	0
Bran Flakes™, breakfast cereal	74	½ cup	18	13
Bran muffin, small	60	3.5 oz	41	25
Brandy	[0]	1 oz	0	0
Brazil nuts	[0]	1.75 oz	0	0
Breton wheat crackers	67	6 crackers	14	10
Broad beans	79	½ cup	11	9
Broccoli, raw	[0]	1 cup	0	0
Broken rice, white, cooked	86	1 cup	43	37
Brown rice, cooked	50	1 cup	33	16
Buckwheat	54	¾ cup	30	16
Bulgur, cooked 20 min	48	¾ cup	26	12
Bun, hamburger	61	1.5 oz	22	13
Butter beans, canned	31	⅔ cup	20	6
C				
Cabbage, raw	[0]	1 cup	0	0
Cactus Nectar, Organic Agave, light, 90% fructose (Western Commerce)	11	1 Tbsp	8	1
Cactus Nectar, Organic Agave, light, 97% fructose (Western Commerce)	10	1 Tbsp	8	1
Cantaloupe, fresh	65	4 oz	6	4
Cappellini pasta, cooked	45	1½ cups	45	20
Carrot juice, fresh	43	8 oz	23	10
Carrots, peeled, cooked	49	½ cup	5	2
Carrots, raw	47	1 medium	6	3
Cashew nuts, salted	22	1.75 oz	13	3
Cauliflower, raw	[0]	¾ cup	0	0
Celery, raw	[0]	2 stalks	0	0
Cheese	[0]	4 oz	0	0

[0] indicates that the food has so little carbohydrate that the GI value cannot be tested. The GL, therefore, is 0.

FOOD	GI Value	Nominal Serving Size	Net Carb per Serving	GL per Serving
Cherries, fresh	22	18	12	3
Chicken nuggets, frozen	46	4 oz	16	7
Chickpeas, canned	42	⅔ cup	22	9
Chickpeas, dried, cooked	28	⅔ cup	30	8
Chocolate cake made from mix with chocolate frosting	38	4 oz	52	20
Chocolate milk, low-fat	34	8 oz	26	9
Chocolate mousse, 2% fat	31	½ cup	22	7
Chocolate powder, dissolved in water	55	8 oz	16	9
Chocolate pudding, made from powder and whole milk	47	½ cup	24	11
Choice DM™, nutritional support product, vanilla (Mead Johnson)	23	8 oz	24	6
Clif® bar (cookies & cream)	101	2.4 oz	34	34
Coca Cola®, soft drink	53	8 oz	26	14
Cocoa Puffs™, breakfast cereal	77	1 cup	26	20
Complete™, breakfast cereal	48	1 cup	21	10
Condensed milk, sweetened	61	2½ Tbsps	27	17
Converted rice, long-grain, cooked 20-30 min, Uncle Ben's®	50	1 cup	36	18
Converted rice, white, cooked 20-30 min, Uncle Ben's®	38	1 cup	36	14
Corn Flakes™, breakfast cereal	92	1 cup	26	24
Corn Flakes™, Honey Crunch, breakfast cereal	72	¾ cup	25	18
Corn pasta, gluten-free	78	1¼ cups	42	32
Corn Pops™, breakfast cereal	80	1 cup	26	21
Corn Thins, puffed corn cakes, gluten-free	87	1 oz	20	18
Corn, sweet, cooked	60	½ cup	18	11
Cornmeal, cooked 2 min	68	1 cup	13	9
Couscous, cooked 5 min	65	¾ cup	35	23

[0] indicates that the food has so little carbohydrate that the GI value cannot be tested. The GL, therefore, is 0.

FOOD	GI Value	Nominal Serving Size	Net Carb per Serving	GL per Serving
Cranberry juice cocktail	52	8 oz	31	16
Crispix™, breakfast cereal	87	1 cup	25	22
Croissant, medium	67	2 oz	26	17
Cucumber, raw	[0]	¾ cup	0	0
Cupcake, strawberry-iced, small	73	1.5 oz	26	19
Custard apple, raw, flesh only	54	4 oz	19	10
Custard, homemade	43	½ cup	26	11
Custard, prepared from powder with whole milk, instant	35	½ cup	26	9

D

FOOD	GI Value	Nominal Serving Size	Net Carb per Serving	GL per Serving
Dates, dried	50	7	40	20
Desiree potato, peeled, cooked	101	5 oz	17	17
Doughnut, cake type	76	1.75 oz	23	17

E

FOOD	GI Value	Nominal Serving Size	Net Carb per Serving	GL per Serving
Eggs, large	[0]	2	0	0
Enercal Plus™ (Wyeth-Ayerst)	61	8 oz	40	24
English Muffin™ bread (Natural Ovens)	77	1 oz	14	11
Ensure™, vanilla drink	48	8 oz	34	16
Ensure™ bar, chocolate fudge brownie	43	1.4 oz	20	8
Ensure Plus™, vanilla drink	40	8 oz	47	19
Ensure Pudding™, old-fashioned vanilla	36	4 oz	26	9

F

FOOD	GI Value	Nominal Serving Size	Net Carb per Serving	GL per Serving
Fanta®, orange soft drink	68	8 oz	34	23
Fettuccine, egg, cooked	32	1½ cups	46	15
Figs, dried	61	3	26	16
Fish	[0]	4 oz	0	0
Fish sticks	38	3.5 oz	19	7
Flan/crème caramel	65	½ cup	73	47
French baguette, white, plain	95	1 oz	15	15

[0] indicates that the food has so little carbohydrate that the GI value cannot be tested. The GL, therefore, is 0.

FOOD	GI Value	Nominal Serving Size	Net Carb per Serving	GL per Serving
French fries, frozen, reheated in microwave	75	30 pcs	29	22
French green beans, cooked	[0]	½ cup	0	0
French vanilla cake made from mix, with vanilla frosting	42	4 oz	58	24
French vanilla ice cream, premium, 16% fat	38	½ cup	14	5
Froot Loops™, breakfast cereal	69	1 cup	26	18
Frosted Flakes™, breakfast cereal	55	1 cup	26	15
Fructose, pure	19	1 Tbsp	10	2
Fruit cocktail, canned, light syrup	55	½ cup	16	9
Fruit leather	61	2 pcs	24	15
G				
Gatorade™ (orange) sports drink	89	8 oz	15	13
Gin	[0]	1 oz	0	0
Glucerna™, vanilla (Abbott)	31	8 oz	23	7
Glucose (dextrose)	99	1 Tbsp	10	10
Glucose tablets	102	3 pcs	15	15
Gluten-free corn pasta	78	1½ cups	42	32
Gluten-free multigrain bread	79	1 oz	13	10
Gluten-free rice and corn pasta	76	1½ cups	49	37
Gluten-free spaghetti, rice and split pea, canned in tomato sauce	68	8 oz	27	19
Gluten-free split pea and soy pasta shells	29	1½ cups	31	9
Gluten-free white bread, sliced	80	1 oz	15	12
Glutinous (sticky) rice, white, cooked	92	⅔ cup	48	44
Gnocchi	68	6 oz	48	33
Grapefruit, fresh, medium	25	1 half	11	3
Grapefruit juice, unsweetened	48	8 oz	20	9
Grape-Nuts® (Post), breakfast cereal	75	¼ cup	21	16

[0] indicates that the food has so little carbohydrate that the GI value cannot be tested. The GL, therefore, is 0.

FOOD	GI Value	Nominal Serving Size	Net Carb per Serving	GL per Serving
Grapes, black, fresh	59	¾ cup	18	11
Grapes, green, fresh	46	¾ cup	18	8
Green peas	48	⅓ cup	7	3
Green pea soup, canned	66	8 oz	41	27
H				
Hamburger bun	61	1.5 oz	22	13
Happiness™ (cinnamon, raisin, pecan bread) (Natural Ovens)	63	1 oz	14	9
Hazelnuts	[0]	1.75 oz	0	0
Healthy Choice™ Hearty 100% Whole Grain	62	1 oz	14	9
Healthy Choice™ Hearty 7-Grain	55	1 oz	14	8
Heary Oatmeal cookies, FIFTY50	30	4 cookies	20	6
Honey	55	1 Tbsp	18	10
Honey graham crackers	74	9 squares	18 squares	13
Hot cereal, apple & cinnamon, dry (ConAgra)	37	1.2 oz	22	8
Hot cereal, unflavored, dry (ConAgra)	25	1.2 oz	19	5
Hunger Filler™, whole-grain bread (Natural Ovens)	59	1 oz	13	7
I				
Ice cream, low-fat, vanilla, "light"	50	½ cup	9	5
Ice cream, premium, French vanilla, 16% fat	38	½ cup	14	5
Ice cream, premium, "ultra chocolate," 15% fat	37	½ cup	14	5
Ice cream, regular fat	61	½ cup	20	12
Instant potato, mashed	97	¾ cup	20	17
Instant rice, white, cooked 6 min	74	¾ cup	42	36
Ironman PR® bar, chocolate	39	2.3 oz	26	10

[0] indicates that the food has so little carbohydrate that the GI value cannot be tested. The GL, therefore, is 0.

FOOD	GI Value	Nominal Serving Size	Net Carb per Serving	GL per Serving
J				
Jam, apricot fruit spread, reduced sugar	55	1½ Tbsps	13	7
Jam, strawberry	51	1½ Tbsps	20	10
Jasmine rice, white, cooked	109	1 cup	42	46
Jelly beans	78	10 large	28	22
K				
Kaiser roll	73	1 half	16	12
Kavli™ Norwegian crispbread	71	5 pcs	16	12
Kidney beans, canned	52	⅔ cup	17	9
Kidney beans, cooked	23	⅔ cup	25	6
Kiwi fruit	53	4 oz	12	7
Kudos® Whole Grain Bars, chocolate chip	62	1.8 oz	32	20
L				
Lactose, pure	46	1 Tbsp	10	5
Lamb	[0]	4 oz	0	0
Leafy vegetables (spinach, arugula, etc.), raw	[0]	1½ cups	0	0
L.E.A.N Fibergy™ bar, Harvest Oat	45	1.75 oz	29	13
L.E.A.N Life long Nutribar™, Chocolate Crunch	32	1.5 oz	19	6
L.E.A.N Life long Nutribar™, Peanut Crunch	30	1.5 oz	19	6
L.E.A.N Nutrimeal™, drink powder, Dutch Chocolate	26	8 oz	13	3
Lemonade, reconstituted	66	8 oz	20	13
Lentil soup, canned	44	9 oz	21	9
Lentils, brown, cooked	29	¾ cup	18	5
Lentils, green, cooked	30	¾ cup	17	5
Lentils, red, cooked	26	¾ cup	18	5

[0] indicates that the food has so little carbohydrate that the GI value cannot be tested. The GL, therefore, is 0.

FOOD	GI Value	Nominal Serving Size	Net Carb per Serving	GL per Serving
Lettuce	[0]	4 leaves	0	0
Life Savers®, peppermint candy	70	18 pcs	30	21
Light rye bread	68	1 oz	14	10
Lima beans, baby, frozen	32	¾ cup	30	10
Linguine pasta, thick, cooked	46	1½ cups	48	22
Linguine pasta, thin, cooked	52	1½ cups	45	23
Long-grain rice, cooked 10 min	61	1 cup	36	22
Lychees, canned in syrup, drained	79	4 oz	20	16

M

FOOD	GI Value	Nominal Serving Size	Net Carb per Serving	GL per Serving
M & M's®, peanut	33	15 pcs	17	6
Macadamia nuts	[0]	1.75 oz	0	0
Macaroni and cheese, made from mix	64	1 cup	51	32
Macaroni, cooked	47	1¼ cups	48	23
Maltose	105	1 Tbsp	10	11
Mango	51	4 oz	15	8
Maple syrup, pure Canadian	54	1 Tbsp	18	10
Marmalade, orange	48	1½ Tbsps	20	9
Mars Bar®	68	2 oz	40	27
Melba toast, Old London	70	6 pcs	23	16
METRx® bar (vanilla)	74	3.6 oz	50	37
Milk Arrowroot™ cookies	69	5	18	12
Millet, cooked	71	⅔ cup	36	25
Mini Wheats™, whole-wheat breakfast cereal	58	12 pcs	21	12
Mousse, butterscotch, 1.9% fat	36	1.75 oz	10	4
Mousse, chocolate, 2% fat	31	1.75 oz	11	3
Mousse, hazelnut, 2.4% fat	36	1.75 oz	10	4
Mousse, mango, 1.8% fat	33	1.75 oz	11	4
Mousse, mixed berry, 2.2% fat	36	1.75 oz	10	4
Mousse, strawberry, 2.3% fat	32	1.75 oz	10	3

[0] indicates that the food has so little carbohydrate that the GI value cannot be tested. The GL, therefore, is 0.

FOOD	GI Value	Nominal Serving Size	Net Carb per Serving	GL per Serving
Muesli bar containing dried fruit	61	1 oz	21	13
Muesli bread, made from mix in bread oven (ConAgra)	54	1 oz	12	7
Muesli, gluten-free, with low-fat milk	39	1 oz	19	7
Muesli, Swiss Formula	56	1 oz	16	9
Muesli, toasted	43	1 oz	17	7
Multi-Grain 9-Grain bread	43	1 oz	14	6
N				
Navy beans, canned	38	5 oz	31	12
Nesquik™, chocolate dissolved in low-fat milk, no-sugar-added	41	8 oz	11	5
Nesquik™, strawberry dissolved in low-fat milk, no-sugar-added	35	8 oz	12	4
New creamer potato, canned	65	5 oz	18	12
New creamer potato, unpeeled and cooked 20 min	78	5 oz	21	16
Noodles, instant "two-minute" (Maggi®)	46	1½ cups	40	19
Noodles, mung bean (Lungkow beanthread), dried, cooked	39	1½ cups	45	18
Noodles, rice, fresh, cooked	40	1½ cups	39	15
Nutella®, chocolate hazelnut spread	33	1 Tbsp	12	4
Nutrigrain™, breakfast cereal	66	1 cup	15	10
Nutty Natural™, whole-grain bread (Natural Ovens)	59	1 oz	12	7
O				
Oat bran, raw	55	2 Tbsp	5	3
Oatmeal, cooked 1 min	66	1 cup	26	17
Oatmeal cookies	55	4 small	21	12
Oatmeal cookies, Sugar-Free, Fifty50	47	4 cookies	28	10

[0] indicates that the food has so little carbohydrate that the GI value cannot be tested. The GL, therefore, is 0.

FOOD	GI Value	Nominal Serving Size	Net Carb per Serving	GL per Serving
Orange juice, unsweetened, reconstituted	53	8 oz	18	9
Orange, fresh, medium	42	4 oz	11	5
P				
Pancakes, buckwheat, gluten-free, made from mix	102	2 4" pancakes	22	22
Pancakes, made from mix	67	2 4" pancakes	58	39
Papaya, fresh	59	4 oz	8	5
Parsnips	97	½ cup	12	12
Pastry	59	2 oz	26	15
Pea soup, canned	66	8 oz	41	27
Peach, canned in heavy syrup	58	½ cup	26	15
Peach, canned in light syrup	52	½ cup	18	9
Peach, fresh, large	42	4 oz	11	5
Peanuts	14	1.75 oz	6	1
Pear halves, canned in natural juice	43	½ cup	13	5
Pear, fresh	38	4 oz	11	4
Peas, green, frozen, cooked	48	½ cup	7	3
Pecans	[0]	1.75 oz	0	0
Pepper, fresh, green or red	[0]	3 oz	0	0
Pineapple, fresh	66	4 oz	10	6
Pineapple juice, unsweetened	46	8 oz	34	15
Pinto beans, canned	45	⅔ cup	22	10
Pinto beans, dried, cooked	39	¾ cup	26	10
Pita bread, white	57	1 oz	17	10
Pizza, cheese	60	1 slice	27	16
Pizza, Super Supreme, pan (11.4% fat)	36	1 slice	24	9
Pizza, Super Supreme, thin and crispy (13.2% fat)	30	1 slice	22	7
Plums, fresh	39	2 medium	12	5
Pop Tarts™, double chocolate	70	1.8 oz pastry	36	25

[0] indicates that the food has so little carbohydrate that the GI value cannot be tested. The GL, therefore, is 0.

FOOD	GI Value	Nominal Serving Size	Net Carb per Serving	GL per Serving
Popcorn, plain, cooked in microwave oven	72	1½ cups	11	8
Pork	[0]	4 oz	0	0
Potato chips, plain, salted	54	2 oz	21	11
Potato, baked	85	5 oz	30	26
Potato, microwaved	82	5 oz	33	27
Pound cake (Sara Lee)	54	2 oz	28	15
PowerBar® (chocolate)	57	2.3 oz	42	24
Premium soda crackers	74	5 crackers	17	12
Pretzels	83	1 oz	20	16
Prunes, pitted	29	6	33	10
Pudding, instant, chocolate, made with whole milk	47	½ cup	24	11
Pudding, instant, vanilla, made with whole milk	40	½ cup	24	10
Puffed crispbread	81	1 oz	19	15
Puffed rice cakes, white	82	3 cakes	21	17
Puffed Wheat, breakfast cereal	80	2 cups	21	17
Pumpernickel rye kernel bread	41	1 oz	12	5
Pumpkin	75	3 oz	4	3

R

FOOD	GI Value	Nominal Serving Size	Net Carb per Serving	GL per Serving
Raisin Bran™, breakfast cereal	61	½ cup	19	12
Raisins	64	½ cup	44	28
Ravioli, meat-filled, cooked	39	6.5 oz	38	15
Red wine	[0]	3.5 oz	0	0
Red-skinned potato, peeled and microwaved on high for 6–7.5 min	79	5 oz	18	14
Red-skinned potato, peeled, boiled 35 min	88	5 oz	18	16
Red-skinned potato, peeled, mashed	91	5 oz	20	18

[0] indicates that the food has so little carbohydrate that the GI value cannot be tested. The GL, therefore, is 0.

FOOD	GI Value	Nominal Serving Size	Net Carb per Serving	GL per Serving
Resource Diabetic™, nutritional support product, vanilla (Novartis)	34	8 oz	23	8
Rice and corn pasta, gluten-free	76	1½ cups	49	37
Rice bran, extruded	19	1 oz	14	3
Rice cakes, white	78	3 cakes	21	17
Rice Krispies™, breakfast cereal	82	1¼ cups	26	22
Rice Krispies Treat™ bar	63	1 oz	24	15
Rice noodles, fresh, cooked	40	1½ cups	39	15
Rice, parboiled	72	1 cup	36	26
Rice pasta, brown, cooked 16 min	92	1½ cups	38	35
Rice vermicelli	58	1½ cups	39	22
Rolled oats	42	1 cup	21	9
Roll-Ups®, processed fruit snack	99	1 oz	25	24
Roman (cranberry) beans, fresh, cooked	46	¾ cup	18	8
Russet, baked potato	85	5 oz	30	26
Rutabaga, fresh, cooked	72	5 oz	10	7
Rye bread	58	1 oz	14	8
Ryvita® crackers	69	3 crackers	16	11

S

FOOD	GI Value	Nominal Serving Size	Net Carb per Serving	GL per Serving
Salami	[0]	4 oz	0	0
Salmon	[0]	4 oz	0	0
Sausages, fried	28	3.5 oz	3	1
Scones, plain	92	1 oz	9	8
Sebago potato, peeled, cooked	87	5 oz	17	14
Seeded rye bread	55	1 oz	13	7
Semolina, cooked (dry)	55	⅓ cup	50	28
Shellfish (shrimp, crab, lobster, etc.)	[0]	4 oz	0	0
Sherry	[0]	2 oz	0	0
Shortbread cookies	64	1 oz	16	10

[0] indicates that the food has so little carbohydrate that the GI value cannot be tested. The GL, therefore, is 0.

FOOD	GI Value	Nominal Serving Size	Net Carb per Serving	GL per Serving
Shredded Wheat™, breakfast cereal	75	⅔ cup	20	15
Shredded Wheat™ biscuits	62	1 oz	18	11
Skim milk	32	8 oz	13	4
Skittles®	70	45 pcs	45	32
Smacks™, breakfast cereal	71	¾ cup	23	11
Smoothie, raspberry (ConAgra)	33	8 oz	41	14
Snack bar, Apple Cinnamon (ConAgra)	40	1.75 oz	29	12
Snack bar, Peanut Butter & Choc-Chip (ConAgra)	37	1.75 oz	27	10
Snickers® bar	68	2.2 oz	35	23
Social Tea Biscuits	55	6 cookies	19	10
Soda crackers, Premium	74	5 crackers	17	12
Soft drink, Coca Cola®	53	8 oz	26	14
Soft drink, Fanta®, orange	68	8 oz	34	23
Sourdough rye	48	1 oz	12	6
Sourdough wheat	54	1 oz	14	8
Soy & Flaxseed bread (mix in bread oven) (ConAgra)	50	1 oz	10	5
Soybeans, canned	14	1 cup	6	1
Soybeans, dried, cooked	20	1 cup	6	1
Spaghetti, durum wheat, cooked 20 min	64	1½ cups	43	27
Spaghetti, gluten-free, rice and split pea, canned in tomato sauce	68	8 oz	27	19
Spaghetti, white, cooked 5 min	38	1½ cups	48	18
Spaghetti, whole wheat, cooked 5 min	32	1½ cups	44	14
Special K™, breakfast cereal	69	1 cup	21	14
Spirali pasta, durum wheat, al dente	43	1½ cups	44	19
Split pea and soy pasta shells, gluten-free	29	1½ cups	31	9
Split pea soup	60	1 cup	27	16

[0] indicates that the food has so little carbohydrate that the GI value cannot be tested. The GL, therefore, is 0.

FOOD	GI Value	Nominal Serving Size	Net Carb per Serving	GL per Serving
Split peas, yellow, cooked 20 min	32	¾ cup	19	6
Sponge cake, plain	46	2 oz	36	17
Squash, raw	[0]	⅔ cup	0	0
Star pastina, white, cooked 5 min	38	1½ cups	48	18
Stay Trim™, whole-grain bread (Natural Ovens)	70	1 oz	15	10
Stoned Wheat Thins	67	14 crackers	17	12
Strawberries, fresh	40	4 oz	3	1
Strawberry jam	51	1½ Tbsps	20	10
Strawberry shortcake	42	2.2 oz	40	17
Stuffing, bread	74	1 oz	21	16
Sucrose	68	1 Tbsp	10	7
Super Supreme pizza, pan (11.4% fat)	36	1 slice	24	9
Super Supreme pizza, thin and crispy (13.2% fat)	30	1 slice	22	7
Sushi, salmon	48	3.5 oz	36	17
Sweet corn, whole kernel, canned, diet-pack, drained	46	1 cup	28	13
Sweet potato, cooked	44	5 oz	25	11

T

FOOD	GI Value	Nominal Serving Size	Net Carb per Serving	GL per Serving
Taco shells, baked	68	2 shells	12	8
Tapioca, cooked with milk	81	¾ cup	18	14
Tofu-based frozen dessert, chocolate with high-fructose (24%) corn syrup	115	1.75 oz	9	10
Tomato juice, canned, no added sugar	38	8 oz	9	4
Tomato soup	38	1 cup	17	6
Tortellini, cheese	50	6.5 oz	21	10
Tortilla chips, plain, salted	63	1.75 oz	26	17
Total™, breakfast cereal	76	¾ cup	22	17
Tuna	[0]	4 oz	0	0
Twix® Cookie Bar, caramel	44	2 cookies	39	17

[0] indicates that the food has so little carbohydrate that the GI value cannot be tested. The GL, therefore, is 0.

FOOD	GI Value	Nominal Serving Size	Net Carb per Serving	GL per Serving
U				
Ultra chocolate ice cream, premium, 15% fat	37	½ cup	14	5
Ultracal™ with fiber (Mead Johnson)	40	8 oz	29	12
V				
Vanilla cake made from mix, with vanilla frosting	42	4 oz	58	24
Vanilla pudding, instant, made with whole milk	40	½ cup	24	10
Vanilla wafers, creme-filled, Fifty50	41	4 cookies	20	8
Vanilla wafers	77	6 cookies	18	14
Veal	[0]	4 oz	0	0
Vermicelli, white, cooked	35	1½ cups	44	16
W				
Waffles, Aunt Jemima®	76	1 4" waffle	13	10
Walnuts	[0]	1.75 oz	0	0
Water crackers	78	7 crackers	18	14
Watermelon, fresh	72	4 oz	6	4
Weet-Bix™, breakfast cereal	69	2 biscuits	17	12
Wheaties™, breakfast cereal	82	1 cup	21	17
Whiskey	[0]	1 oz	0	0
White bread	70	1 oz	14	10
White rice, instant, cooked 6 min	87	1 cup	42	36
White wine	[0]	3.5 oz	0	0
100% Whole Grain™ bread (Natural Ovens)	51	1 oz	13	7
Whole milk	31	8 oz	12	4
Whole-wheat bread	77	1 oz	12	9
Wonder™ white bread	80	1 oz	14	11

[0] indicates that the food has so little carbohydrate that the GI value cannot be tested. The GL, therefore, is 0.

FOOD	GI Value	Nominal Serving Size	Net Carb per Serving	GL per Serving
X				
Xylitol	8	1 Tbsp	10	1
Y				
Yam, peeled, cooked	37	5 oz	36	13
Yogurt, low-fat, wild strawberry	31	8 oz	34	11
Yogurt, low-fat, with fruit and artificial sweetener	14	8 oz	15	2
Yogurt, low-fat, with fruit and sugar	33	8 oz	35	12

[0] indicates that the food has so little carbohydrate that the GI value cannot be tested. The GL, therefore, is 0.

◀ 20 ▶

LOW TO HIGH GI VALUES

*F*OR THOSE WHO wish to choose a diet with the lowest GI values possible, we've created the following listing in order of GI values (i.e., from lowest to highest value). We've also divided the list into food categories, so that when you want to find a low-GI vegetable or fruit, for example, the information is at your fingertips. The categories are:

- bakery products
- beverages
- breads
- breakfast foods
- cookies
- crackers
- dairy products and alternatives
- fruits and fruit products
- grains
- infant formulas and baby foods

- legumes
- meal-replacement products
- mixed meals and convenience foods
- noodles
- pasta
- protein foods
- snack foods and candy
- soups
- special dietary products
- sugars
- vegetables

As we discuss in *The New Glucose Revolution*, it's not necessary to eat all of your carbohydrates from low-GI sources. If half of your carbohydrate choices have low GI values, you're doing well. If you also eat a low-GI food at each meal, you'll be reducing the GI values overall.

FOOD	LOW	INTERMEDIATE	HIGH

BAKERY PRODUCTS

Cakes

FOOD	LOW	INTERMEDIATE	HIGH
Banana	○		
Chocolate, with chocolate frosting	○		
Pound	○		
Sponge	○		
Vanilla	○		
Angel food		◑	
Flan		◑	

Muffins

FOOD	LOW	INTERMEDIATE	HIGH
Apple with sugar or artificial sweeteners	○		
Apple, oat, and raisin	○		
Banana, oat, and honey		◑	
Bran		◑	
Blueberry		◑	
Carrot		◑	
Oatmeal, made from mix, Quaker Oats		◑	
Cupcake, iced			●
Scone, plain			●

Pastries

FOOD	LOW	INTERMEDIATE	HIGH
Croissant		◑	
Doughnut, cake-type			●

BEVERAGES

Alcoholic

FOOD	LOW	INTERMEDIATE	HIGH
Beer	○		
Brandy	○		

FOOD	LOW	INTERMEDIATE	HIGH
Gin	○		
Sherry	○		
Whiskey	○		
Wine, red	○		
Wine, white	○		
Juices			
Apple, with sugar or artificial sweetener	○		
Carrot, fresh	○		
Grapefruit, unsweetened	○		
Pineapple, unsweetened	○		
Tomato, canned, no added sugar	○		
Smoothies and shakes			
Raspberry	○		
Soy	○		
Soft drinks			
Coca-Cola®		◑	
Fanta®		◑	
Sports drinks			
Gatorade®			●

BREADS

Fruit			
Muesli, made from mix	○		
Happiness™, cinnamon, raisin, pecan		◑	
Gluten-free			
Fiber-enriched			●
White			●

FOOD	LOW	INTERMEDIATE	HIGH
Rye			
Pumpernickel	○		
Sourdough	○		
Cocktail		◐	
Light		◐	
Whole-wheat		◐	
Spelt			
Multigrain	○		
White			●
Wheat			
100% Whole Grain	○		
Soy & Linseed bread machine mix	○		
Flatbread, Indian		◐	
Hearty 7 Grain		◐	
Pita, plain		◐	
Bagel			●
Baguette			●
Bread stuffing			●
English muffin			●
Flatbread, Middle Eastern			●
Italian			●
Lebanese, white			●
White, enriched			●
Whole-wheat			●

FOOD	LOW	INTERMEDIATE	HIGH

BREAKFAST FOODS

Breakfast cereal bars

FOOD	LOW	INTERMEDIATE	HIGH
Rice Krispies® Treat		◐	

Cooked cereals

FOOD	LOW	INTERMEDIATE	HIGH
Hot cereal, apple & cinnamon, ConAgra	○		
Old-fashioned oats	○		
Cream of Wheat™, regular, Nabisco		◐	
One Minute Oats, Quaker Oats		◐	
Quick Oats, Quaker Oats		◐	
Cream of Wheat™, instant, Nabisco			●
Oatmeal, instant			●

Grain products

FOOD	LOW	INTERMEDIATE	HIGH
Pancakes, prepared from mix	○		
Pancakes, buckwheat, gluten-free, made from mix			●
Waffles, Aunt Jemima®			●

Ready-to-eat cereals

FOOD	LOW	INTERMEDIATE	HIGH
All-Bran®, Kellogg's	○		
Complete™ Bran Flakes, Kellogg's	○		
Bran Buds™, Kellogg's		◐	
Bran Chex™, Kellogg's		◐	
Froot Loops™, Kellogg's		◐	
Frosted Flakes™, Kellogg's		◐	
Just Right™, Kellogg's		◐	
Life™, Quaker Oats		◐	
Nutrigrain™, Kellogg's		◐	
Oat bran, raw, Quaker Oats		◐	
Puffed Wheat, Quaker Oats		◐	

FOOD	LOW	INTERMEDIATE	HIGH
Raisin Bran™, Kellogg's		◐	
Special K™, Kellogg's		◐	
Bran Flakes™, Kellogg's			●
Cheerios™, General Mills			●
Corn Chex™, Kellogg's			●
Corn Flakes™, Kellogg's			●
Corn Pops™, Kellogg's			●
Grapenuts™, Post			●
Rice Krispies™, Kellogg's			●
Shredded Wheat™, Nabisco			●
Team™ Flakes, Nabisco			●
Total™			●
Weetabix™			●

COOKIES

FOOD	LOW	INTERMEDIATE	HIGH
Hearty Oatmeal, FiFTY50	○		
Oatmeal, Sugar-Free, FiFTY50	○		
Vanilla wafers, creme filled, FiFTY50	○		
Arrowroot		◐	
Digestives		◐	
Tea biscuits		◐	
Shortbread		◐	
Vanilla wafers			●

CRACKERS

FOOD	LOW	INTERMEDIATE	HIGH
Breton wheat		◐	
Melba toast		◐	
Rye crispbread		◐	
Ryvita™		◐	
Stoned Wheat Thins		◐	
Water		◐	

FOOD	LOW	INTERMEDIATE	HIGH
Kavli™ Norwegian Crispbread			●
Premium soda (Saltines)			●
Rice cakes, puffed			●

DAIRY PRODUCTS AND ALTERNATIVES

Custard

Homemade	O		

Ice cream

Regular	O		

Milk

Low-fat, chocolate, with aspartame	O		
Low-fat, chocolate, with sugar	O		
Skim	O		
Whole	O		
Condensed, sweetened			●

Mousse

Butterscotch, low-fat, Nestlé	O		
Chocolate, low-fat, Nestlé	O		
French vanilla, low-fat, Nestlé	O		
Hazelnut, low-fat, Nestlé	O		
Mango, low-fat, Nestlé	O		
Mixed berry, low-fat, Nestlé	O		
Strawberry, low-fat, Nestlé	O		

Pudding

Instant, chocolate, made with milk	O		
Instant, vanilla, made with milk	O		

FOOD	LOW	INTERMEDIATE	HIGH
Soy milk			
Reduced-fat	O		
Whole	O		
Soy yogurt			
Tofu-based frozen dessert, chocolate			●
Yogurt			
Low-fat, fruit, with aspartame	O		
Low-fat, fruit, with sugar	O		
Nonfat, French vanilla, with sugar	O		
Nonfat, strawberry, with sugar	O		

FRUIT AND FRUIT PRODUCTS

FOOD	LOW	INTERMEDIATE	HIGH
Apple, fresh	O		
Apricot, fresh	O		
Banana, fresh	O		
Cantaloupe, fresh	O		
Cherries, fresh	O		
Grapefruit, fresh	O		
Grapes, fresh	O		
Kiwi, fresh	O		
Mango, fresh	O		
Orange, fresh	O		
Peach, canned in natural juice	O		
Peach, fresh	O		
Pear, canned in pear juice	O		
Pear, fresh	O		
Plum, fresh	O		
Prunes, pitted	O		
Strawberries, fresh	O		
Strawberry jam	O		
Figs, dried		◑	

FOOD	LOW	INTERMEDIATE	HIGH
Fruit cocktail, canned		◐	
Papaya, fresh		◐	
Peach, canned in heavy syrup		◐	
Peach, canned in light syrup		◐	
Pineapple, fresh		◐	
Raisins/sultanas		◐	
Dates, dried			●
Lychee, canned in syrup, drained			●
Watermelon, fresh			●

GRAINS

FOOD	LOW	INTERMEDIATE	HIGH
Barley, cracked	○		
Barley, pearled	○		
Buckwheat	○		
Buckwheat groats	○		
Bulgur	○		
Corn, canned, no salt added	○		
Rice, brown	○		
Rice, Cajun Style, Uncle Ben's®	○		
Rice, Long Grain and Wild, Uncle Ben's®	○		
Rice, parboiled, converted, white, cooked 20–30 min, Uncle Ben's®	○		
Barley, rolled		◐	
Corn, fresh		◐	
Cornmeal		◐	
Couscous		◐	
Rice, arborio (risotto)		◐	
Rice, Basmati		◐	
Rice, Garden Style, Uncle Ben's®		◐	
Rice, parboiled, long-grain, cooked 10 minutes		◐	
Millet			●

FOOD	LOW	INTERMEDIATE	HIGH
Rice, sticky			●
Rice, parboiled			●
Tapioca boiled with milk			●

INFANT FORMULA AND BABY FOODS

Baby foods

	LOW	INTERMEDIATE	HIGH
Apple, apricot, and banana, baby cereal		◐	
Chicken and noodles with vegetables, strained		◐	
Corn and rice, baby		◐	
Oatmeal, creamed, baby		◐	
Rice pudding, baby		◐	

Infant formula

	LOW	INTERMEDIATE	HIGH
SMA, 20 cal./fl oz, Wyeth	○		
Nursoy, soy-based, milk-free, Wyeth		◐	

LEGUMES

Beans

	LOW	INTERMEDIATE	HIGH
Baked, canned	○		
Butter, dried and cooked	○		
Kidney, canned	○		
Lima, baby, frozen	○		
Mung, cooked	○		
Navy, dried and cooked	○		
Pinto, cooked	○		
Soy, canned	○		

Lentils

	LOW	INTERMEDIATE	HIGH
Green, dried and cooked	○		
Red, dried and cooked	○		

FOOD	LOW	INTERMEDIATE	HIGH
Peas			
Black-eyed	○		
Chickpeas/garbanzo beans, canned	○		
Split, yellow, cooked	○		

MEAL-REPLACEMENT PRODUCTS

	LOW	INTERMEDIATE	HIGH
Designer chocolate, sugar-free, Worldwide Sport Nutrition low-carbohydrate products	○		
L.E.A.N Fibergy™ bar, Harvest Oat, Usana	○		
L.E.A.N (Life long) Nutribar™, Peanut Crunch, Usana	○		
L.E.A.N (Life long) Nutribar™, Chocolate Crunch, Usana	○		

MIXED MEALS and CONVENIENCE FOODS

	LOW	INTERMEDIATE	HIGH
Chicken nuggets, frozen, reheated	○		
Fish fillet, reduced fat, breaded	○		
Fish sticks	○		
Greek lentil stew with a bread roll, homemade	○		
Lean Cuisine™, chicken with rice	○		
Pizza, Super Supreme, pan, Pizza Hut	○		
Pizza, Super Supreme, thin and crispy, Pizza Hut	○		
Pizza, Vegetarian Supreme, thin and crispy, Pizza Hut	○		
Spaghetti Bolognese	○		
Sushi, salmon	○		
Tortellini, cheese, Stouffer	○		
Tuna patty, reduced fat	○		
Cheese sandwich, white bread		◑	
Kugel		◑	
Macaroni and cheese, boxed, Kraft		◑	
Peanut-butter sandwich, white/whole-wheat bread		◑	
Pizza, cheese, Pillsbury		◑	

FOOD	LOW	INTERMEDIATE	HIGH
Spaghetti, gluten-free, canned in tomato sauce		◐	
Sushi, roasted sea algae, vinegar and rice		◐	
Taco shells, cornmeal-based, baked, El Paso		◐	
White bread and butter		◐	
Stir-fried vegetables with chicken and rice, homemade			●

NOODLES

Instant	○		
Mung bean, Lungkow beanthread	○		
Rice, fresh, cooked	○		
Rice, dried, cooked		◐	
Udon, plain, reheated 5 min		◐	

PASTA

Capellini	○		
Fettuccine, egg	○		
Gluten-free, cornstarch	○		
Linguine, thick, fresh, durum wheat, white	○		
Linguine, thin, fresh, durum wheat	○		
Macaroni, plain, cooked	○		
Ravioli	○		
Spaghetti, cooked 5 min	○		
Spaghetti, cooked 22 min	○		
Spaghetti, protein-enriched, cooked 7 min	○		
Spaghetti, whole-wheat	○		
Spirali, cooked, durum wheat	○		
Star pastina, cooked 5 min	○		
Tortellini	○		
Vermicelli	○		
Gnocchi		◐	

FOOD	LOW	INTERMEDIATE	HIGH
Rice vermicelli		◐	
Spaghetti, cooked 10 min, Barilla		◐	
Corn, gluten-free			●
Rice and corn, gluten-free			●
Rice, brown, cooked 16 min			●

PROTEIN FOODS

FOOD	LOW	INTERMEDIATE	HIGH
Beef	○		
Cheese	○		
Cold cuts	○		
Eggs	○		
Fish	○		
Lamb	○		
Pork	○		
Sausages	○		
Shellfish (shrimp, crab, lobster, etc.)	○		
Veal	○		

SNACK FOODS AND CANDY

Candy

FOOD	LOW	INTERMEDIATE	HIGH
Nougat	○		
Jelly beans			●
Life Savers®			●
Skittles®			●

Chips

FOOD	LOW	INTERMEDIATE	HIGH
Corn, plain, salted, Doritos™	○		
Potato, plain, salted	○		

Chocolate bars

FOOD	LOW	INTERMEDIATE	HIGH
Milk, Cadbury's	○		

FOOD	LOW	INTERMEDIATE	HIGH
Milk, Dove®, Mars	○		
Milk, Nestlé	○		
White, Milky Bar®	○		
Mars Bar®		◑	
Snickers Bar®		◑	
Chocolate candy			
M & M's®, peanut	○		
Chocolate spread			
Nutella®, chocolate hazelnut spread	○		
Dried-fruit bars			
Fruit Roll-Ups®			●
Nuts			
Cashews	○		
Peanuts	○		
Pecans	○		
Popcorn			
Plain, microwaved			●
Pretzels			
Plain, salted			●
Snack bars			
Apple Cinnamon, ConAgra	○		
Peanut Butter & Choc-Chip	○		
Twix® Cookie Bar, caramel	○		
Kudos Whole Grain Bars, chocolate chip		◑	
Sports bars			
Ironman PR bar®, chocolate	○		

FOOD	LOW	INTERMEDIATE	HIGH
PowerBar®, chocolate		◑	

SOUPS

FOOD	LOW	INTERMEDIATE	HIGH
Lentil, canned	○		
Minestrone, canned, ready-to-serve	○		
Tomato, canned	○		
Black bean, canned		◑	
Green pea, canned		◑	
Split pea, canned		◑	

SPECIAL DIETARY PRODUCTS

FOOD	LOW	INTERMEDIATE	HIGH
Choice DM™, vanilla, Mead Johnson	○		
Ensure™, Abbott	○		
Ensure Plus™, vanilla, Abbott	○		
Ensure Pudding™, vanilla, Abbott	○		
Ensure™ bar, chocolate fudge brownie, Abbott	○		
Ensure™, vanilla, Abbott	○		
Glucerna™ bar, lemon crunch, Abbott	○		
Glucerna™ SR shake, vanilla, Abbott	○		
Glucerna™, vanilla, Abbott	○		
Resource Diabetic™, vanilla, Novartis	○		
Resource Plus, chocolate, Novartis	○		
Ultracal™ with fiber, Mead Johnson	○		
Enercal Plus™, Wyeth-Ayerst		◑	
Enrich Plus shake, vanilla, Ross		◑	

SUGARS

FOOD	LOW	INTERMEDIATE	HIGH
Blue Agave, Organic Agave Cactus Nectar, light, 90% fructose, Western Commerce	○		
Blue Agave, Organic Agave Cactus Nectar, light, 97% fructose, Western Commerce	○		
Fructose	○		

FOOD	LOW	INTERMEDIATE	HIGH
Lactose	○		
Honey		◑	
Sucrose		◑	
Glucose			●
Maltose			●

VEGETABLES

FOOD	LOW	INTERMEDIATE	HIGH
Artichokes	○		
Avocado	○		
Bok choy	○		
Broccoli	○		
Cabbage	○		
Carrots, peeled, cooked	○		
Cassava (yucca), cooked with salt	○		
Cauliflower	○		
Celery	○		
Corn, canned, no salt added	○		
Cucumber	○		
French beans (runner beans)	○		
Leafy greens	○		
Lettuce	○		
Peas, frozen, cooked	○		
Pepper	○		
Potato, sweet	○		
Squash	○		
Yam	○		
Beet		◑	
Corn, sweet, cooked		◑	
Potato, boiled/canned		◑	
Potato, new, canned		◑	
Taro		◑	

FOOD	LOW	INTERMEDIATE	HIGH
Broad beans			●
Parsnips			●
Potato, French fries, frozen and reheated			●
Potato, instant			●
Potato, mashed			●
Potato, microwaved			●
Potato, russet, baked			●
Pumpkin			●
Rutabaga			●

GLYCEMIC INDEX TESTING

*I*F YOU ARE a food manufacturer, you may be interested in having the glycemic index of some of your products tested on a fee-for-service basis. For more information, contact:

Sydney University Glycaemic Index Research Service
(SUGiRS)
Department of Biochemistry
University of Sydney
NSW 2006 Australia
Fax: (61) (2) 9351-6022
E-mail: j.brandmiller@staff.usyd.edu.au

FOR MORE INFORMATION

To find a dietitian:

The American Dietetic Association
120 S. Riverside Plaza
Suite 2000
Chicago, IL 60606
Phone: 1-800-877-1600
www.eatright.org

To order Natural Ovens bread:

Natural Ovens Bakery
PO Box 730
Manitowoc, WI 54221
Phone: 1-800-772-0730
www.naturalovens.com

ACKNOWLEDGMENTS

WE WOULD LIKE to acknowledge the extraordinary efforts of Johanna Burani and Linda Rao, who adapted this book—and the other books in *The New Glucose Revolution Pocket Guide* series—for North American readers. Together they have worked to ensure that every piece of information is accurate and appropriate for readers in the United States and Canada.

ABOUT THE AUTHORS

HELEN O'CONNOR, B.Sc., DIP. N.D., PH.D., is a sports dietitian and lecturer in the Department of Exercise and Sport Science at the University of Sydney. O'Connor consults at the Sydney Sports Medicine Centre, Olympic Park, and at South Sydney Sports Medicine Centre. She is a consultant dietitian to the Sydney Swans, Canterbury Rugby League, and a number of Australia's elite athletes.

■

JENNIE BRAND-MILLER, PH.D., is a Professor of Human Nutrition in the Human Nutrition Unit at the University of Sydney and President of the Nutrition Society of Australia. Professor Brand-Miller was awarded the prestigious Clunies Ross National Science and Technology Medal for her work on nutrition and the management of blood sugar.

■

STEPHEN COLAGIURI, M.D., is the President of the Australian Diabetes Society, director of the Diabetes Center, and head of the Department of Endocrinology, Metabolism, and Diabetes at the Prince of Wales Hospital, Randwick, New South Wales, Australia. He is a graduate of the University of Sydney (M.B.B.S., 1970) and a member of the Royal Australasian College of Physicians (1977). He has joint academic appointments at the University of New South Wales. He has authored more than 100 scientific papers, many concerned with the importance of carbohydrate in the diet of people with diabetes. A co-author of The Glucose Revolution and several other titles in The Glucose Revolution Pocket Guide Series, he lives in Sydney, Australia.

■

KAYE FOSTER-POWELL, B.SC.,M. NUTR. & DIET., is an accredited practicing dietitian with extensive experience in diabetes management. She has conducted research into the glycemic index of foods and its practical applications over the last 15 years. Currently she is a dietitian with Wentworth Area Diabetes Services and provides consultancy on all aspects of the glycemic index.

■

LINDA RAO, M.ED., a freelance writer and editor, has been writing and researching health topics for the past 16 years. Her work has appeared in several national publications, including *Prevention, Organic Style,* and *Better Homes & Gardens.* She serves as a contributing editor for *Prevention* magazine and is the co-adapter, with Johanna Burani, of all the titles in *The Glucose Revolution* Pocket Guide Series. She lives in Allentown, Pennsylvania.

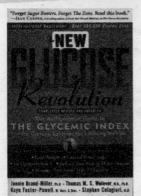
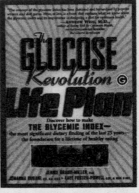

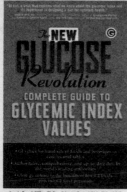

THE NEW GLUCOSE REVOLUTION COMPLETE GUIDE TO GLYCEMIC INDEX VALUES

The *Only* Authoritative, Comprehensive, Up-to-Date Guide to Glycemic Index Values—A Companion to *The New Glucose Revolution*

With GI values for hundreds of foods and beverages, *The New Glucose Revolution Complete Guide to Glycemic Index Values* makes it easier than ever to ascertain a food's GI value. Each of the three easy-to-read tables in this book lists a food's GI value, serving size, net carbohydrate per serving, and glycemic load, which is clearly explained.

WHAT MAKES MY BLOOD GLUCOSE GO UP . . . AND DOWN?

And 101 Other Frequently Asked Questions About Your Blood Glucose Levels

In this accessible, informative book, *The New Glucose Revolution*'s Jennie Brand-Miller and Kaye Foster-Powell team up with leading diabetes journalist Rick Mendosa to answer the most frequently asked questions about your blood glucose levels, from "What is a normal blood glucose level?" to "What should I eat when I crave something sweet?"

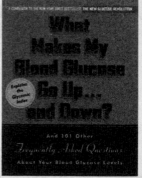

THE NEW GLUCOSE REVOLUTION COMPLETE GUIDE TO LOSING WEIGHT

The *Only* Authoritative Guide to Losing Weight Using the Glycemic Index—A Companion to *The New Glucose Revolution*

Learn how you can best use the glycemic index for effective weight loss. *The New Glucose Revolution Pocket Guide to Losing Weight* clearly describes the differences between carbohydrates and how low-GI foods can help you feel fuller longer, burn more body fat, and achieve and maintain a healthy weight and lifelong eating habits.

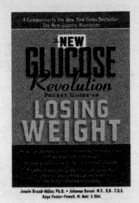

ISBN 1-56924-498-7 • $6.95

THE NEW GLUCOSE REVOLUTION COMPLETE GUIDE TO GLYCEMIC DIABETES

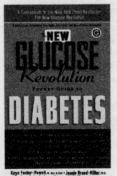

The *Only* Authoritative Guide to Managing Diabetes Using the Glycemic Index— A Companion to *The New Glucose Revolution*

Get the most up-to-date information about using the GI to manage type 1 and type 2 diabetes. This informative guide clearly explains which types of carbohydrate are best to eat and offers practical tips on how to use the GI to control your blood glucose throughout the day.

ISBN 1-5692-499-5 • $6.95

THE NEW GLUCOSE REVOLUTION POCKET GUIDE TO THE TOP 100 LOW GI FOODS

The *Only* Authoritative Guide to the Top 100 Low GI Foods—A Companion to *The New Glucose Revolution*

This handy A to Z guide offers in-depth entries for the top 100 foods with the lowest GI values. It covers each food's nutritional benefit and includes GI values, glycemic load, carbohydrate, fiber and fat content, plus handy eating tips and a low-GI Food Finder.

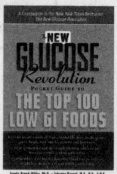

ISBN 1-5692-500-2 • $6.95

THE NEW GLUCOSE REVOLUTION POCKET GUIDE TO THE METABOLIC SYNDROME AND YOUR HEART

The *Only* Authoritative Guide to Using the Glycemic Index for Better Heart Health—A Companion to *The New Glucose Revolution*

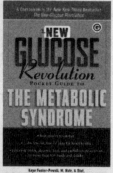

Get the most up-to-date information about using the glycemic index to keep your heart healthy and reduce your risk of having a heart attack. This book explains the importance of slowly digested, low-GI carbohydrates and provides important heart-related dietary guidelines for managing your blood glucose levels, controlling insulin sensitivity, and losing weight.

ISBN 1-56924-449-9 • $6.95

Food manufacturers are showing increasing interest in having the GI values of their products measured. Some are already including the GI value of foods on food labels. As more and more research highlights the benefits of low-GI foods, consumers and dietitians are writing and telephoning food companies and diabetes organizations asking for GI data. This symbol has been registered in several countries, including the United States and Australia, to indicate that a food has been properly GI tested—in real people, not in a test tube—and also makes a positive contribution to nutrition. You can find out more about the program at www.gisymbol.com.au.

As consumers, you have a right to information about the nutrients and physiological effects of foods. You have a right to know the GI value of a food and to know it has been tested using appropriate standardized methodology.